Machine Learning and Python for Human Behavior, Emotion, and Health Status Analysis

This book is a practical guide for individuals interested in exploring and implementing smart home applications using Python. Comprising six chapters enriched with hands-on codes, it seamlessly navigates from foundational concepts to cutting-edge technologies, balancing theoretical insights and practical coding experiences. In short, it is a gateway to the dynamic intersection of Python programming, smart home technology, and advanced machine learning applications, making it an invaluable resource for those eager to explore this rapidly growing field.

Key Features:

- Throughout the book, practicality takes precedence, with hands-on coding examples accompanying each concept to facilitate an interactive learning journey.

- Striking a harmonious balance between theoretical foundations and practical coding, the book caters to a diverse audience, including smart home enthusiasts and researchers.

- The content prioritizes real-world applications, ensuring readers can immediately apply the knowledge gained to enhance smart home functionalities.

- Covering Python basics, feature extraction, deep learning, and XAI, the book provides a comprehensive guide, offering an overall understanding of smart home applications.

Machine Learning and Python for Human Behavior, Emotion, and Health Status Analysis

Written by
Md Zia Uddin

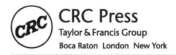

CRC Press
Taylor & Francis Group
Boca Raton London New York

CRC Press is an imprint of the
Taylor & Francis Group, an **informa** business

Designed cover image: Freepik

First edition published 2025
by CRC Press
2385 NW Executive Center Drive, Suite 320, Boca Raton FL 33431

and by CRC Press
4 Park Square, Milton Park, Abingdon, Oxon, OX14 4RN

CRC Press is an imprint of Taylor & Francis Group, LLC

© 2025 Md Zia Uddin

ISBN: 978-1-032-54478-6 (hbk)
ISBN: 978-1-032-54635-3 (pbk)
ISBN: 978-1-003-42590-8 (ebk)

DOI: 10.1201/9781003425908

Typeset in Minion
by SPi Technologies India Pvt Ltd (Straive)

Contents

Preface

This book is a practical guide to smart home applications using Python, divided into six chapters with hands-on codes. It starts with an introduction and covers Python basics in the second chapter. Chapter 3 explores pulling important info from data through feature extraction techniques, and then Chapter 4 dives into machine learning and Explainable AI (XAI). The exciting part of the book is to be found in Chapters 5 and 6. Chapter 5 presents real-life examples of behavior and health analysis using deep learning and XAI. Then, the final chapter explores recognizing emotions through cameras and audio using deep learning and XAI. The book strikes a balance between theory and practical coding, making it accessible for both smart home enthusiasts and researchers. A little glimpse of each chapter follows:

The opening chapter introduces the topic of smart homes and machine learning, shedding light on diverse projects. It explores various smart home initiatives, showcasing the seamless integration of technology into daily life. A central focus is the pivotal role of machine learning in data extraction and analysis. Machine learning tools emerge as transformative, aiding caregivers and clinical experts in diagnosis and decision-making. The chapter unravels insights into the impact of these projects on healthcare and caregiving landscapes, laying the groundwork for a deeper understanding of the symbiotic relationship between smart homes and machine learning. Readers embark on a journey where innovative technologies not only enhance our homes but also revolutionize the delivery of healthcare. This chapter sets the stage for a comprehensive exploration, promising a deeper dive into the fascinating fusion of smart living and machine intelligence.

Chapter 2 focuses on Python and its libraries, with a number of real-world examples. It starts with the basics of Python, in order to ensure that everyone feels comfy and ready for the journey. We learn about things like variables, data types, and making choices in our code. It's like building the ABCs of Python! This part is great for beginners because lots of hands-on activities are there to really understand how Python works. It then jumps into some cool libraries, which are like special tools that make Python even more awesome. It then checks out NumPy for doing math stuff, Pandas for playing with data, Matplotlib for creating cool charts, and Seaborn for even fancier visualizations. Each library is explained with real examples, so it's not just theory—you get to see how these tools can solve real problems. By the end of this chapter, you'll know the ABCs of Python and have some nifty tools in your coding backpack. It's like starting with the basics to build a strong foundation for all the cool things discussed in the next chapters.

Chapter 3 dives into the world of feature extraction techniques using Python—PCA, Kernel PCA (KPCA), Independent Component Analysis (ICA), and Linear Discriminant Analysis (LDA). It's like uncovering secrets to refine data in machine learning! With Python, PCA steals the spotlight, making data simpler by capturing the important stuff and reducing complexity. KPCA takes it a step further, smoothly handling tricky nonlinear data structures. Then, it explores ICA, pulling out hidden factors in the data by focusing on independent components. LDA steps up with Python demos, showing off its skill in boosting supervised learning by making classes more distinct. These techniques are not just theoretical—they get down to real-world applications like image processing, signal analysis, and text mining. The chapter proves how adaptable and useful these techniques are across different fields. By using them, machine learning models become champs at spotting important patterns.

Chapter 4 unfolds the world of deep learning and explainable AI. Recently, researchers have been drawn to deep learning techniques for modeling patterns in input data, with Convolutional Neural Networks (CNN) gaining popularity for its superior discriminative power compared to previous approaches. CNN, a type of deep learning, involves feature extractions and convolutional stacks to build a hierarchy of abstract features. For time-sequential event analysis, Recurrent Neural Networks like long short-term memory (LSTM) shine, offering strong discriminative power. Enter Neural Structured Learning (NSL), an advanced open-source framework within deep learning algorithms designed to grasp events in data. NSL leverages structured signals tied to feature inputs, employing neural graph learning to train networks based on graphs and structured data. It extends basic adversarial learning by utilizing structured data with valuable relational information among samples. Acknowledging the remarkable strides in Artificial Intelligence (AI), the chapter addresses the challenge of explainability (XAI) arising amid AI success. It explores various machine learning techniques—both shallow and deep—alongside XAI algorithms, navigating the dynamic landscape of AI advancements and challenges.

Chapter 5 is packed with cool stories showing how wearable sensors, machine learning, and explainable AI (XAI) can be combined in real-life situations. First up is behavior recognition—it's like teaching computers to understand how people act using wearable sensors and smart learning. They look at public datasets to figure out and explain what our actions mean. Next, it jumps into real-time activity recognition. Imagine your fitness tracker not just counting steps but instantly knowing if you're running, walking, or doing yoga. That's the magic of wearable sensors and machine learning working together, making our gadgets super-smart. The tech adventure continues with real-time body skeleton tracking using cameras that can see both color and heat. It's like having a virtual map of how people move in real time, opening doors for lots of cool applications. Heading home, we explore real-time home monitoring and behavior prediction. Ambient sensors keep an eye on what's happening, and machine learning predicts what might happen next. It's like having a super-smart home that understands your routines. Health takes the spotlight next with predictions about oxygen levels and pulse using wearable sensors. It's not just about tracking—it's also predicting, and thereby making health monitoring more personalized and efficient. We wrap up the tech journey with real-time respiration prediction, where ultra-wideband sensors and machine learning team up to give instant and accurate predictions, taking healthcare to a whole new level. In a nutshell, Chapter 5 is all about real stories where technology, smart sensors, and intelligent machine learning work together to understand our behavior, predict activities, monitor our homes, and even take health monitoring to new heights.

Chapter 6 takes us into the world of recognizing emotions, first through cameras and then using audio. With cameras, it explores different features like Principal Component Analysis (PCA), Independent Component Analysis (ICA), and Local Directional Patterns (LDP), teaming up with machine learning to understand facial expressions and emotions in pictures. The chapter doesn't stop there—it goes into real-time emotion recognition, making things even more exciting. To help us understand how the computer makes these predictions, it introduces Explainable AI (XAI). Moving on to audio-based emotion recognition, the chapter introduces Mel-Frequency Cepstral Coefficients (MFCC) as special features to capture emotions in sound. Different machine learning algorithms join the party to decode the emotional vibes hidden in spoken words or audio signals. In a nutshell, the chapter unfolds a journey where technology learns to recognize emotions, in terms of both pictures and also what we say. It's not just about understanding technical details; it's about seeing how these smart systems can grasp and respond to human emotions. Whether it's decoding smiles on camera or sensing emotions in our voice, this chapter shows us the exciting possibilities of machines understanding how we feel.

Acknowledgments

To my beloved wife (Syeda Farzana Zerin) and children (Zayan Adeeb and Fayzan Aabid), your relentless support, love, and encouragement have been the guiding forces on my journey. You are my inspiration, my motivation, and my greatest treasures.

To my dear parents (Ahmed Sharif and Monoara Begum), your love, sacrifices, and commitments have shaped me into the person I am today.

This book is dedicated to you all, as a token of my deepest gratitude and appreciation.

Author

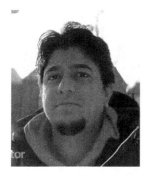

Md Zia Uddin was born in 1981 at Haji Alimuddin's House, 18 No Ward, East Bakalia, Chittagong, Bangladesh. He is the youngest child of Ahmed Sharif (Late) and Monoara Begum. Dr. Zia completed his PhD in Biomedical Engineering in 2011. He is currently working as a Senior Research Scientist in Sustainable Communication Technologies department of SINTEF Digital, Oslo, Norway. SINTEF is the largest research institute in Scandinavia and one of the largest research institutes in Europe. He has been leading/working on work packages of various national and international research projects. His research fields are mainly focused on data and feature analysis from various sources for physical/mental healthcare using machine learning/artificial intelligence/XAI. Dr. Zia also has a good teaching experience with more than 20 computer science-related courses from bachelor's degree to PhD.

Dr. Zia Uddin has got more than 150 peer-reviewed research publications including prestigious international journals, conferences, and book chapters. Half of the publications are led or mostly done by him. His google scholar citations are around 4500. He got Gold Medal Award (2008) for academic excellence in undergraduate study. He was also Awarded Korean Government IT Scholarship (March 2007 to February 2011) and Kyung Hee University President Scholarship (March 2007 to February 2011). His research works received best/outstanding paper awards in several peer reviewed international conferences. He acted as a reviewer in many prestigious journals including IEEE Transactions on Pattern Analysis and Machine Intelligence (TPAMI), Information Fusion, IEEE Transactions on Industrial Informatics, and IEEE Transactions on Biomedical Engineering, etc.

Dr. Zia Uddin has been leading/working in different work packages of national and international research projects. He has been enlisted in the World's Top 2% Scientists since 2019, conducted by Stanford University of USA and Elsevier BV. For more information about his work and background: https://sites.google.com/site/webpagezia/home

## CHAPTER 1

Smart Assisted Homes, Sensors, and Machine Learning

1.1 SMART HOMES

A smart home, or a connected or automated home, is a dwelling equipped with the latest technology and built with systems and devices that can be interconnected to make your life easier and more comfortable [1–3]. Examples are the Internet of Things (IoT), artificial intelligence (AI), and various communication technologies that have combined to pave the way for smart homes. So, an integrated and connected smart home is an integrated and controlled environment that allows the control, monitoring, and automation of various devices and systems. It is often possible to manage and optimize living spaces through the Internet or a local network, a capability once considered inconceivable for homeowners. The concept of smart homes has traversed a remarkable evolutionary journey. It commenced with rudimentary automation features such as programmable thermostats and remote-controlled garage doors. Today, smart homes have become sophisticated ecosystems due to the rapid advancement of technology, particularly in the Internet of Things (IoT) and AI. The significance of smart homes extends beyond mere convenience. They are designed to address the practical needs and challenges of contemporary living. These connected spaces aim to enhance comfort, energy efficiency, security, and the overall quality of life. Moreover, smart homes contribute to broader societal goals, such as sustainable living and improved healthcare. The foundation of smart homes lies in a synergy of cutting-edge technologies that enable seamless integration and intelligent control. Understanding these technologies is crucial to grasping the essence of smart homes.

DOI: 10.1201/9781003425908-1

1.1.1 Technologies

At the heart of smart homes is the Internet of Things (IoT), a vast network of interconnected physical objects equipped with sensors, software, and coy features. IoT devices collect and communicate data over the Internet or other networks, forming the basis for smart home functionality. AI, specifically machine learning, is the brainpower behind smart homes. Machine learning algorithms empower devices to learn from user behavior, adapt to preferences, and make intelligent decisions. Voice assistants like Amazon's Alexa and Google Assistant are prime examples of AI in action. Effective communication between devices is essential in a smart home ecosystem. Various communication protocols, such as Wi-Fi, Zigbee, and Z-Wave, facilitate seamless data exchange, ensuring devices can work together harmoniously. Sensors, ranging from motion detectors to temperature sensors, gather environmental data. Actuators, like motors or switches, execute actions based on this data. For instance, smart thermostats use temperature sensors to regulate heating and cooling, enhancing comfort and energy efficiency. Voice assistants have become the central interface in many smart homes. They utilize natural language processing to understand and respond to voice commands, serving as the command centers for controlling a wide array of smart devices. A smart home's ecosystem comprises various components, each contributing to the overall functionality and experience. Let's explore the key elements that define a modern smart home. Smart appliances encompass a range of household machines, including refrigerators, ovens, washing machines, and dishwashers. What sets them apart is their connectivity and ability to be remotely controlled and monitored. These appliances often feature energy-saving modes and can even provide notifications when maintenance is required. Intelligent lighting systems offer homeowners complete control over their lighting environments. Users can adjust brightness, color, and scheduling to create custom lighting scenarios. Automation capabilities enable lights to adapt based on time of day or occupancy, enhancing energy efficiency and security.

Smart thermostats have redefined heating and cooling management in homes. They learn user preferences, adapt to daily routines, and optimize temperature settings for comfort and energy savings. They can be controlled remotely via smartphone apps, ensuring a comfortable environment upon arrival. Security is a top priority for homeowners, and intelligent security systems provide advanced solutions. These systems include intelligent cameras, smart doorbells, motion sensors, and locks. With remote monitoring and real-time alerts, homeowners can enhance security and peace of mind. Voice assistants, such as Amazon's Alexa and Google Assistant, have become integral to many smart homes. They serve as the central control hubs for various devices, responding to voice commands to control lighting, music, thermostats, and more. Smart TVs and speakers offer access to extensive entertainment options, from streaming services to music and games. Voice control simplifies content access and navigation, providing a seamless and immersive entertainment experience. Smart homes increasingly incorporate health and wellness devices, catering to residents' well-being. These devices include fitness trackers, smart scales, air quality monitors, and connected medical devices. They empower individuals to monitor and manage their health from the comfort of their homes. Energy management systems tie together various devices and sensors to optimize energy usage. Homeowners can track energy consumption, receive insights, and make informed decisions to reduce their carbon footprint and utility bills. Home automation hubs serve as centralized controllers for diverse smart devices. They enable automation, scheduling, and remote control, offering a single interface for managing the entire smart home ecosystem.

1.1.2 Benefits

Smart homes bring numerous advantages to homeowners, enhancing their living experiences. Let's explore the key benefits that have made smart homes increasingly popular. The most apparent benefit of smart homes is their unparalleled convenience. Homeowners can effortlessly automate daily tasks, adjust settings, and control devices with a simple tap on a smartphone or a voice command. From adjusting lighting to regulating temperature, smart homes prioritize user comfort. Smart homes are designed to be energy-efficient. Smart thermostats and lighting systems optimize energy usage, lowering utility bills. Moreover, they contribute to reducing the overall carbon footprint, aligning with sustainability goals. Security is a paramount concern for homeowners, and smart homes address this with advanced solutions. Surveillance cameras, motion sensors, and smart locks provide real-time monitoring and immediate alerts, bolstering home security. Innovative entertainment systems offer access to vast content and entertainment options. With voice-controlled interfaces, users can navigate their favorite shows, movies, and music, creating an immersive and enjoyable entertainment experience.

Health and wellness devices within smart homes enable individuals to take charge of their well-being. Fitness trackers, for instance, track physical activity, while air quality monitors ensure a healthy living environment. The ability to remotely monitor and control smart homes is a game-changer. Whether adjusting the thermostat while at work or checking security cameras while on vacation, homeowners can stay connected to their residences, enhancing security and convenience. While the initial investment in smart home technology can be substantial, long-term savings from reduced energy consumption, improved maintenance, and enhanced security often outweigh the upfront costs.

1.1.3 Challenges

Despite their numerous advantages, smart homes also present a set of challenges and concerns that homeowners and manufacturers must address to ensure a secure and seamless experience. The interconnected nature of smart homes raises concerns about privacy and data. Unauthorized access to devices or data breaches can compromise sensitive information. Implementing robust security measures, such as encryption and regular software updates, is essential to mitigate these risks. Not all smart devices are compatible, which can lead to interoperability issues. This can frustrate homeowners who desire a seamless experience across their devices and ecosystems. The upfront costs of purchasing and installing smart devices can hinder adoption for some homeowners. However, it's essential to consider the long-term savings and benefits when evaluating these costs. Setting up and configuring a smart home ecosystem can be complex, often requiring technical expertise. Manufacturers are working to simplify installation, but it remains challenging for some users. Smart devices rely on stable internet connections, and if the network goes down, some functionalities may be lost. Additionally, vulnerabilities in device firmware or software can be exploited by cybercriminals. The rapid pace of technological advancement means that devices can become obsolete quickly. This can be frustrating for homeowners who invest in innovative technology only to find it outdated within a few years. While smart homes can contribute to energy savings, producing electronic devices can have environmental consequences. Sustainable practices and responsible disposal are essential to mitigate this impact. Smart homes are vulnerable to various cyberattacks, including unauthorized access to devices, data breaches, and the possibility of devices being used as entry points into home networks. Understanding these risks is crucial for homeowners. Ensuring that only authorized users can control and access smart devices is vital. Multi-factor authentication and secure user accounts are essential for a secured smart home. Manufacturers must implement secure device management practices. This includes regularly issuing firmware updates to patch vulnerabilities and address security issues promptly.

Homeowners can take proactive steps to enhance the security of their smart homes. This includes regularly updating device firmware, using strong and unique passwords, segmenting the network, and exercising caution when granting access to third-party apps and services.

1.2 EXAMPLE SMART ASSISTED HOMES

Smart assisted homes are designed to assist users based on sensors and other technologies such as machine learning. The growing number of older adults generates a significant demand for healthcare services. Age is a vital risk factor for the development of chronic disorders. Older adults also have a substantial risk of falling. One of the significant problems in handling this complex care is that resources are becoming more abundant daily [3, 4]. Through recent advances in sensor and communication technologies, monitoring technologies have become essential for achieving a robust healthcare system that can help older adults live independently for a longer time [5, 6].

Among the researchers of smart care systems for assisted living, many of them focused on developing smart older adult care systems that could observe interactions between older adults and their living environment over a long period [7–16]. Such user behavioral monitoring systems for older people use different smart devices such as magnetic switches to record movement in rooms, infrared sensors to detect activities, and sound sensors to determine the types of activities. Thus, the system could respond to any activity outside standard activity patterns. Other technologies emerged in the following decades that focused on monitoring elderly behaviors such as daily activities and fall detection. However, an overview of non-wearable ambient sensor-based systems would be valuable for analyzing the increasingly complicated care demands of older adults.

During the last few decades, many researchers have tried to carry out smart home projects. For instance, GatorTech [17] is an earlier smart home project developed at the University of Florida. The project adopted various ambient sensors to provide several user services, such as voice and behavior recognition. The CASAS project [18] was a smart home project that was carried out at Washington State University in 2007. It was a multi-disciplinary project for developing a smart home using different sensors and actuators.

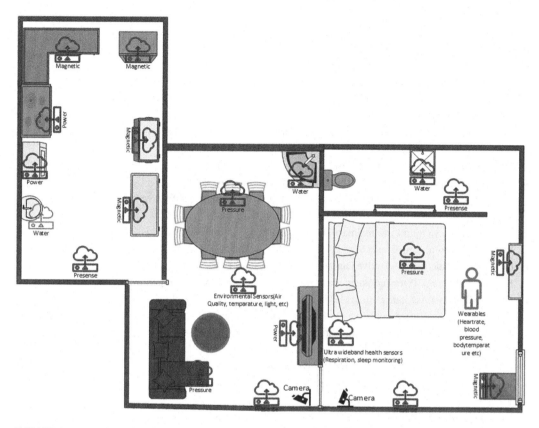

FIGURE 1.1   An example of a smart home of a user's residence.

The researchers in the project adopted machine learning tools for user behavior analysis. They focused on creating a lightweight design that could be easily set up without further customization. SWEET-HOME was a French project on developing a smart home system primarily based on audio technology [19]. The project aimed at three key goals: developing an audio-based interactive technology that gives users complete control over the home environment. Figure 1.1 shows an example of a smart home with sensors installed in different places.

1.3 EVENTS IN SMART ASSISTED HOMES

In recent years, several applications for diabetes control, depression treatment, hypertension control, medication adherence, and psychological support have been developed to allow people to live alone while having the possibility of daily control over their health status. Alarm-alerting applications can save human life when critical events, such as falls, prolonged inactivity, or environmental dangers, are detected. The early detection of behavioral changes is necessary before a notable deterioration of the primary activities involved in daily living. Scientific studies have pointed out that people's activity levels drop significantly when they retire. By the early identification of the risk factors of functional decline, this can be prevented in a large portion of the elderly population at the time of retirement by targeting timely interventions and reducing the risks. Furthermore, behavioral change

TABLE 1.1   List of Possible Events and Devices in Smart Home

Events and Devices for Smart Homes

- Occupancy Detection: Motion Sensors
- Sleep Patterns Monitoring: Wearable Sleep Trackers, Bed-Based Sensors
- Fall Detection: Accelerometers, Gyroscopes
- Medication Reminders: Smart Pill Dispensers
- Health Monitoring: Vital Sign Monitors (e.g., Heart Rate Monitors, Blood Pressure Monitors)
- Daily Routine Assistance: Voice Assistants, Smart Mirrors
- Intruder Detection: Door and Window Sensors, Motion Sensors
- Emergency Response System: Panic Buttons, Wearable Emergency Buttons
- Home Automation Based on Preferences: Smart Thermostats, Smart Lighting Systems
- Social Interaction Facilitation: Video Cameras, Voice Assistants
- Energy Efficiency Optimization: Smart Thermostats, Energy Monitoring Sensors
- Water Usage Monitoring: Smart Water Meters, Water Leak Sensors
- Cognitive Stimulation: Interactive Displays, Cognitive Games
- Exercise and Fitness Tracking: Wearable Fitness Trackers, Smart Exercise Equipment
- Grocery shopping Assistance: Smart Fridges, Barcode Scanners
- Environmental Quality Monitoring: Air Quality Sensors, Humidity Sensors
- Mood Enhancement Smart Lighting Systems, Aromatherapy Diffusers
- Remote Family Connection: Video Cameras, Video Calling Devices
- Routine Maintenance Alerts: Wearable Maintenance Sensors
- Pet Care Assistance: Smart Pet Collars, Pet Activity Trackers
- Posture Correction Reminders: Posture Monitoring Wearables
- Sunlight Exposure Optimization: Smart Blinds, Sunlight Sensors
- Entertainment Recommendations: Smart TVs, Content Recommendation Systems
- Visitor Recognition and Access Control: Facial Recognition Cameras, Smart Door Locks
- Voice-Activated Control Systems: Voice Assistants, Voice Recognition Sensors
- Financial Management Assistance: Smart Budgeting Apps, Expense Trackers
- Personalized Recipe Suggestions: Smart Kitchen Appliances, Recipe Apps
- Learning and Educational Support: Interactive Displays, Educational Apps
- Calendar and Appointment Management: Calendar Apps, Voice Assistants
- Hydration Monitoring: Smart Water Bottles, Hydration Sensors

applications include monitoring dangerous attitudes, such as smoking, calorie intake for diet and exercise, and physical activity levels. Table 1.1 shows the possible list of events.

In assisted living technology-based literature, most researchers have focused on assisted systems for indoor environments. One of the critical application contexts related to medical and public health practices is supported by devices that deliver healthcare services via mobile communication. New technologies and systems have been developed for the continuous monitoring of physical, behavioral, and environmental data and for assessing outcomes from the data. Via the development of systems based on the data from distinguished heterogeneous sensors and additional self-reported data, new information regarding physiological, psychological, emotional, and environmental states can be derived.

Indoor environments can mainly be differentiated into two categories: firstly, homes where people usually live alone or possibly live with a few relatives; secondly, retirement residences where more people live together, move in shared spaces, perform group or individual activities, and undertake controlled physical activities. People's health status can be evaluated by observing their movements, recognizing their actions, evaluating resting periods, monitoring food intake, etc. People's behavioral analysis can be done by detecting anomalies while comparing the actual behavioral events with the expected ones. Besides, social activities in a group and interactions with relatives or friends can also be monitored.

1.4 SENSORS IN SMART HOMES

For different application domains, other technologies can be used to develop assisted living systems, from IoT devices to complex sensor networks consisting of ambient environmental sensors, intelligent devices, video cameras, etc. The variety of sensors or technologies would increase the complexity of data since it can remarkably change in size, heterogeneity, and sampling rates. This section examines the essential technologies for detecting people in assisted living situations.

Devices such as smart objects, wearable sensors, smartwatches, and smartphones are combined with non-invasive sensors such as video cameras or infrared motion sensors, to develop intelligent people monitoring systems for indoor and outdoor applications. The variety of technological systems is quite wide to satisfy particular constraints such as non-invasiveness, subject acceptance, and non-affecting users during everyday activities. In the following, four principal categories of technologies will be examined. Let's start from those that can be easily used, such as wearable sensors, but that require user acceptance, and then move on to those that are less invasive but require structuring objects or furniture, i.e., intelligent everyday objects, up to environmental sensors and social assistive robots. Table 1.2 shows the list of sensors that can be used for smart assisted homes.

1.4.1 Wearable Sensors

The wearable sensor industry has made several advances in miniaturization and energy efficiency in recent years. The most common wearable sensors, usually worn around the hip or wrist, are three-axis accelerometers, gyroscopes, and magnetometers. As well as assessing postural stability, detecting and classifying falls, or analyzing gait cycles, they have been extensively applied to various purposes [20–29]. Further, these sensors are embedded in mobile technologies, such as smartphones, smartwatches, and wristbands, which can also continuously monitor biological, behavioral, and environmental data.

The passive technology of Radio-Frequency Identification (RFID) has been widely employed for identifying dynamic positions in indoor environments by identifying people's dynamic positions. A wearable electromagnetic marker (tag) generating information regarding human motion can be detected by an interrogating antenna that radiates an electromagnetic field that a remote receiver or reader senses. In addition to monitoring movement, location, and even accidental falls, this type of system is also used to detect a fall in the event of an accident.

As far as assisted living systems have been evaluated, they are primarily concerned with monitoring the behavior of residents. To determine an individual's overall health status, several other relevant parameters must also be observed. A physiological parameter is a

TABLE 1.2   List of Sensors in a Smart Home

Sensors for Smart Homes	
• Motion	
• Door/Window	• RFID (Radio-Frequency Identification)
• Contact	• Tilt
• Bed	• Pulse Oximeters
• Pressure /Mat Alarms	• Blood Glucose Monitors
• Occupancy	• Electrocardiogram (ECG)
• Temperature	• Incontinence
• Humidity	• Sound Level
• Cameras	• Touch
• Voice and Sound	• Oxygen Concentration
• Smoke Detectors	• UV-C Disinfection
• Gas Detectors	• Skin Temperature
• Medication Adherence	• Bluetooth Beacons
• Wearable Health Devices	• Air Quality
• Flood	• CO_2
• Leak	• Light
• GPS Trackers	• Water Quality
• Smart Lighting	• Smart Pill Dispensers
• Environmental	• Smart Thermostats
• Weight	• Noise Level
• Proximity	• Blood Pressure Monitors
• Infrared (IR)	• Pulse Rate
• UV Light	

parameter that is measured and referred to as a vital sign. Such parameters include a person's heart rate (HR), blood pressure, temperature, respiration rate, and blood oxygen saturation. For a complete and long-term health monitoring system to be built into everyday scenarios, different sensors can be used to monitor vital bodily functions in addition to the sensors above, which are complementary to each other to monitor critical body functions. There are new possibilities for continuous vital sign monitoring with microelectromechanical systems due to recent advances in performance and cost-effectiveness. Several promising techniques are being explored to extract information on cardiac events and phases, especially ballistocardiography (BCG) and seismocardiography (SCG). In addition to measuring breathing rates and quality metrics of physical activity, they also measure vibrations caused by heart muscle contractions. They are based on IMU sensors placed over the subject's sternum. In addition to smart technology, portable objects, such as glasses, can also be equipped with sensors to monitor some vital signs, including the heart rate and respiration rate, the regularity of pulse and respiration, the occurrence of and duration of apneas, and the distribution of temperature on the face. The use of such techniques is very significant for healthcare professionals, because it allows them to collect necessary information regarding the medical condition of their patients without the use of dedicated hardware, but instead by using more natural methods.

1.4.2 Ambient Sensors

Sensors for environmental monitoring are used to detect parameters that may adversely impact elderly people, such as temperature or air quality. Furthermore, they assist in monitoring daily living activities or localizing individuals and objects around them [30–44]. Environmental sensors are not invasive for people and are not structured or replaced by household objects as opposed to wearable and smart object sensors. It is possible to monitor the different activities of different people through radio frequency-based systems, which analyze the reflections of radio frequency signals. For example, the sleep quality of older adults can be analyzed by inferring the sleeping posture of a subject, capturing people's 3D dynamics, and detecting changes in movement patterns. In addition to operating through optically opaque materials, such as clothing, microwave sensors may eventually detect fog and smoke as they are not affected by external visible lights and scene colours, and they will ultimately be capable of sensing through these materials. It is possible to recognize multiple non-cooperative people's hands and vital signs using intelligent metasurface systems capable of translating microwave data into images. There are several environmental sensory systems that can be utilized to collect biomedical signals, but intelligent optical systems are an example of these systems. These systems can detect rigid and uncontrollable gestures, postural instability, or small tremors, warning signs of neurological conditions. To maintain a healthy lifestyle under observation and notify caregivers during a call for help, low-cost devices such as Kinect, RealSense, and Wii can be easily installed to monitor people's day-to-day activity.

It has been reported that passive infrared (PIR) motion sensors can be used to detect individual movements in research works [45–60]. Usually, PIR motion sensors are heat-sensitive and can detect the presence of users in a room by utilizing temperature changes produced by the sensors. They are installed in the walls of the home of older homes to continuously collect motion data that is related to predefined activities within the sensor's range. A PIR motion sensor can detect various events, such as stove use, temperature changes, water use, and cabinet openings. All of these events can be detected with motion sensors. Motion data can be obtained by a base station that collects data and forwards it to caregivers so that trend analysis can be performed to detect changes in daily activities. Once the data has been gathered, the caregivers can analyze the data and determine what changes have occurred. PIR sensors can also be used to detect changes in health status by using the analysis results. Therefore, they can recognize patterns in daily activities and be triggered as soon as deviations occur to provide alerts. Smart homes can adopt the sensors for various applications, including monitoring the level of activity and detecting falls or other significant events that may occur. An everyday use of monitoring technologies is to detect daily activities and essential events simultaneously so they can be combined to achieve several aims. A PIR motion sensor can also analyze gait velocity, user location, time spent out of the home, sleeping patterns, and nighttime activities. A lot of PIR sensors have been investigated for a wide range of purposes.

For eldercare, video sensors are the most widely used ambient sensors. In ambient assistive living, many studies have been conducted using video cameras to locate and recognize residents within their homes to perform various tasks [61–80]. By removing background from the background, obtaining body shape from the body, analyzing features, and applying machine learning to the data, cameras on walls or ceilings can detect activity. Video-monitoring technology has been utilized primarily to detect activities of daily living, falls, and other significant occurrences.

Among ambient sensors, the Doppler radar is one of the most appealing because it can detect when there is stationary clutter in the background such as a wall [81–83]. As a result of its ability to penetrate intense obstacles, such as furniture items and walls, it achieves a better perception of older adults compared to vision-based sensors. Furthermore, the system does not create any privacy issues when monitoring the home and does not provide the inconvenience of wearables. Moreover, Doppler radar can also be utilized to detect human cardiopulmonary motion, which may offer a promising approach to eliminating the problems of false triggers. Ultra-wideband radar sensors are also prominent candidates for monitoring older adults' occupancy, sleep, and respiration in real time [84–88]. There are many practical applications for the sensor, including monitoring the vital signs of elderly persons, personal security, environmental monitoring, industrial automation, and home automation.

1.5 MACHINE LEARNING

Smart assisted homes are closely related to machine learning since system intelligence is crucial to this research area [89–90]. As a subfield of AI, machine learning focuses on creating algorithms and statistical models that allow computers to enhance their performance in specific tasks by learning from data. Unlike traditional programming, machine learning systems acquire knowledge from data, detect patterns, and make decisions or predictions. Machine learning has gained immense importance across diverse industries, such as healthcare, finance, marketing, and technology. It has revolutionized decision-making, process automation, and insights extraction from large datasets. Its key benefits include automation, predictive analytics, personalization, medical diagnosis, and natural language processing (Table 1.3).

There are four fundamental concepts of machine learning described as follows:

- Data serves as the lifeblood of machine learning, taking forms such as structured data (e.g., tables), unstructured data (e.g., text, images, and audio), and semi-structured data (e.g., JSON, XML). Features represent the variables or attributes in data that models use for predictions. Data preprocessing, encompassing cleaning, normalization, and feature engineering, is a pivotal step in data preparation for machine learning.

- Machine learning models act as mathematical representations of systems or problems learned from data. These models can range from simple linear regression to complex deep neural networks. Algorithms constitute the mathematical techniques used for model training and optimization. Standard algorithms include decision trees, k-nearest neighbors, support vector machines, and gradient boosting.

TABLE 1.3   List of Machine Learning Algorithms

Machine Learning Algorithms

Supervised Learning Algorithms:

- Decision Trees
- Random Forest
- Support Vector Machines (SVM)
- Naive Bayes
- Gradient Boosting Machines
- Linear Regression
- Adaptive Learning Algorithms

Unsupervised Learning Algorithms:

- Clustering Algorithms
- K-Means Clustering
- Hierarchical Clustering
- Anomaly Detection Algorithms
- Hidden Markov Models (HMM)
- K-Nearest Neighbors (KNN)

Deep Learning and Neural Networks:

- Recurrent Neural Networks (RNN)
- Long Short-Term Memory (LSTM)
- Convolutional Neural Networks (CNN)
- Deep Q Networks (DQN)

Transfer Learning Algorithms:

- VGG (Visual Geometry Group)
- ResNet (Residual Networks)
- Inception Networks
- BERT (Bidirectional Encoder Representations from Transformers)
- GPT (Generative Pre-trained Transformer)
- Reinforcement Learning

Explainable Al Algorithms:

- LIME (Local Interpretable Model-agnostic Explanations)
- SHAP (SHapley Additive exPlanations)
- ELI5 (Explain Like I'm 5)
- Anchors (High-Precision Model-Agnostic Explanations)

- Training a machine learning model involves exposing it to labeled data (data with known outcomes) to learn patterns and relationships. Subsequently, model testing on unseen data assesses its performance. Data typically splits into training, validation, and test sets to ensure robust generalization.

- Evaluating a machine learning model's performance is vital to gauge its effectiveness. Standard evaluation metrics include accuracy, precision, recall, F1-score, and mean squared error (MSE) tailored to the problem type (classification, regression, etc.).

1.5.1 Supervised Learning

Supervised learning is one of the most prevalent and utilized machine learning types. In supervised learning, models train on a labeled dataset, where each input data point corresponds to a known output or target [91–92]. The objective is to learn a mapping from input features to the correct output. Supervised learning holds diverse applications across domains, such as

- Identifying objects within images, such as detecting cats or dogs in photographs.
- Tasks like sentiment analysis, text classification, and language translation.
- Predicting disease outcomes, diagnosing medical conditions, and drug discovery.
- Credit scoring, fraud detection, and stock price prediction.
- Offering tailored product recommendations on e-commerce platforms.
- Implementing supervised learning for object detection and decision-making.

Supervised learning is divided into two primary subcategories: classification and regression.

Classification tasks entail assigning input data points to predefined categories or classes. For instance, given an image of a handwritten digit, the goal might be to classify it as one of the digits from 0 to 9. Standard algorithms encompass logistic regression, decision trees, Support Vector Machines, and neural networks.

Regression tasks involve predicting continuous numeric values or quantities. Examples include forecasting house prices based on factors like square footage and location or estimating a person's age based on various demographic variables. Linear regression, polynomial regression, and neural networks apply to regression tasks.

1.5.2 Unsupervised Learning

Unsupervised learning addresses data lacking labels or categorization. In unsupervised learning, algorithms seek patterns, structures, or relationships within data without prior knowledge of these patterns [93, 94]. Unsupervised learning applies across diverse domains:

- Segregating customers with analogous behaviors or preferences for targeted marketing.
- Decreasing image storage space requirements while conserving vital data.
- Identifying rare events or anomalies within data.
- Discovering themes or subjects within textual data.
- Discerning concealed patterns in user behavior for enhanced recommendations.

Unsupervised learning is subdivided into various subtypes:

- Clustering involves grouping similar data points into clusters or categories based on their inherent similarities. Prominent clustering algorithms encompass k-means clustering and hierarchical clustering. Clustering finds utility in customer segmentation, image segmentation, and document clustering.

- Dimensionality reduction techniques strive to reduce data dimensions while preserving essential information. Principal Component Analysis (PCA) and t-distributed Stochastic Neighbor Embedding (t-SNE) are prevalent dimensionality reduction techniques. They support data visualization and feature selection.

- Anomaly detection identifies data points that are significantly divergent from the majority. It proves valuable in scenarios like fraud detection, network security, and manufacturing quality control.

1.5.3 Semi-Supervised Learning

Semi-supervised learning amalgamates elements from supervised and unsupervised learning [95, 96]. In this paradigm, the algorithm receives a small, labeled dataset alongside a more extensive unlabeled dataset. The goal is to enhance model performance using the labeled data. Semi-supervised learning finds relevance in scenarios where obtaining labeled data poses challenges, such as the following.

- Training speech recognition models with limited transcribed audio data.

- Classifying documents when only a subset is labeled.

- Recognizing objects in images with minimal labeled instances.

- Identifying unusual behavior in systems or networks with a limited number of known anomalies.

Semi-supervised learning is a pragmatic middle ground between resource-intensive supervised learning and the complexity of understanding extensive unlabeled data in unsupervised learning. Semi-supervised learning proves exceptionally advantageous when acquiring labeled data is demanding or time-consuming. The labeled data assists in guiding the learning process and optimizing available information. Standard techniques encompass self-training and co-training.

1.6 DEEP MACHINE LEARNING

Deep learning, a subset of machine learning, has profoundly impacted the field of AI [97]. It has completely transformed how machines perceive, learn, and make decisions, resembling human cognition. Deep learning models, particularly neural networks, serve as the foundation of this technological advancement, and their applications span a wide range of domains, from computer vision to natural language processing and beyond. At its core, deep learning revolves around artificial neural networks. These networks draw inspiration from the structure and function of the human brain, featuring layers of interconnected nodes, or neurons, that process and transmit information. The term "deep" in deep learning refers to the multiple layers these networks can possess, allowing them to uncover intricate patterns and representations within raw data.

Deep neural networks are characterized by including numerous hidden layers between the input and output layers. These hidden layers enable the network to acquire intricate and hierarchical data representations. Convolutional Neural Networks (CNNs) and Recurrent Neural Networks (RNNs) are prevalent types of deep neural networks. Deep learning persists as a vibrant and quickly evolving domain, with ongoing research and groundbreaking developments across diverse domains. Deep learning has realized notable advancements across a spectrum of applications:

- CNNs have achieved human-level performance in image classification tasks.

- Transformers, a class of deep neural networks, have transformed NLP tasks, encompassing language translation and chatbots.

- Deep learning has elevated the precision of speech recognition systems.

- Deep neural networks are pivotal for perception and decision-making in self-driving cars.

- Deep learning models support medical image analysis, disease diagnosis, and drug discovery.

The impact of deep learning extends across a multitude of industries. In computer vision, deep neural networks adeptly process visual data, empowering self-driving cars to identify pedestrians, road signs, and other vehicles, thus ensuring safe navigation. In natural language processing (NLP), deep learning models proficiently comprehend and respond to human language, powering chatbots and virtual assistants such as Siri and ChatGPT. Healthcare experiences significant improvements as deep learning aids in disease diagnosis, drug discovery, and the analysis of medical images, ultimately enhancing patient care and outcomes. In the financial sector, deep learning algorithms are at the forefront of fraud detection, algorithmic trading, risk assessment, and safeguarding financial systems. Autonomous vehicles heavily rely on deep learning for navigation, environmental perception, and real-time decision-making, offering a future of safer and more efficient transportation. In robotics, deep learning augments the capabilities of robots, enabling them to execute intricate tasks in unstructured environments. Creative industries harness the power of deep learning to generate art, music, and video content, enriching the world of entertainment and artistic expression.

Nevertheless, deep learning is full of its set of challenges and limitations. One significant challenge is its reliance on copious amounts of labeled data for training, which may only sometimes be readily available for specific tasks or domains. Overfitting poses another issue: models excel in training data but need to improve on unseen data, necessitating the deployment of regularization techniques. The training process for deep neural networks demands substantial computational resources, including the utilization of GPUs or TPUs, and an extensive amount of time. Moreover, the interpretability of deep learning models remains a concern, as they are often regarded as "black boxes," making it arduous to comprehend their decision-making processes. Transfer learning, the knowledge gained from one task to another, only sometimes lends itself to seamless application in deep learning and necessitates judicious model selection and adaptation.

Deep learning continues to evolve, propelled by a slew of promising trends. Research into explainable AI seeks to imbue deep learning models with greater transparency and interpretability, providing insight into their decision-making processes. Federated learning introduces the concept of models being collaboratively trained on decentralized data sources, thus elevating privacy and security. By blending deep learning with reinforcement learning techniques, reinforcement learning enables machines to acquire knowledge and make decisions via interactions with their surroundings. The intersection of quantum computing and deep learning, known as quantum machine learning, holds the potential to solve complex problems exponentially faster. Ethical considerations gain increasing importance, ensuring that deep learning models remain equitable, unbiased, and accountable in their decision-making processes. The following are different deep learning methods used in short.

- Convolutional Neural Networks (CNNs) excel in tasks involving images and grid-like data. They harness convolutional layers to discern features from raw pixel values autonomously. CNNs have demonstrated their mettle in image classification, object detection, and image generation.

- Recurrent Neural Networks (RNNs) are custom-built for sequential data, making them suitable for tasks centered on time series data, NLP, and speech recognition. RNNs boast a recurrent or feedback connection that facilitates the retention of prior inputs.

- Generative Adversarial Networks (GANs) offer a unique approach by orchestrating a face-off between two networks: a generator and a discriminator. GANs find utility in generating fresh data samples, such as images, music, or text, by training the generator to produce indistinguishable contents from genuine data. This innovative technology is extensively employed in art generation, video game design, and special effects.

- Autoencoders are another subset of neural networks adept at unsupervised learning and data compression. Comprising an encoder and a decoder, autoencoders deftly reduce the dimensionality of input data while preserving essential information. They come to the fore in tasks such as image denoising and anomaly detection.

1.6.1 Transfer Learning

Transfer learning emerges as a machine learning technique that leverages knowledge garnered from one task to amplify performance on another related yet distinct task [97–100]. In transfer learning, a model initially trains on a source task and subsequently adapts or fine-tunes for a target task. Transfer learning emerges as an invaluable tool for constructing effective machine learning models under restricted data and computational resources. Transfer learning finds extensive utility across a range of applications:

- Fine-tuning pre-trained CNNs to suit specific image classification tasks.

- Modifying pre-trained language models like BERT for tasks like sentiment analysis or question-answering.

- Harnessing pre-trained models to facilitate medical image analysis and diagnosis.

- Employing transfer learning for tasks including speech recognition and audio classification.

- Leveraging knowledge from one domain to enhance recommendations in another.

Transfer learning frequently commences with a pre-trained model that has already captured valuable features from an extensive dataset, such as a deep neural network trained on an extensive image dataset like ImageNet. These pre-trained models encode general features, including edges, textures, and high-level object representations.

To implement transfer learning, the pre-trained model undergoes adaptation or fine-tuning using a smaller dataset pertinent to the target task. This adaptation process empowers the model to specialize in the target domain's subtleties while retaining the source task's general knowledge.

1.7 LIMITATIONS OF MACHINE LEARNING

It is true that machine learning as a whole, including deep learning, has enabled computers to learn from data, making predictions or decisions without explicit programming. Its applications span various industries, from self-driving cars to medical diagnosis. However, machine learning is not a panacea and comes with limitations and challenges.

1.7.1 Underfitting and Overfitting

Machine learning is a powerful tool for making predictions and decisions based on data. However, when developing machine learning models, it's crucial to balance complexity and simplicity. Two common challenges that arise in this context are underfitting and overfitting. The most common problems in machine learning are these two. Let's dive into these concepts in plain terms, along with real-world examples.

Underfitting occurs when a machine learning model is too simple to capture the underlying patterns in the data. It needs to learn more from the training data to make accurate predictions. Think of it as trying to fit a straight line to a highly nonlinear dataset. Imagine we're trying to predict a person's salary based on their years of experience. We used a linear regression model, which assumes a straight-line relationship between these variables. However, the actual relationship might be curved or nonlinear. In this case, the linear model would underfit the data, resulting in poor predictions.

On the other side of the spectrum, we have overfitting. This happens when a machine learning model is too complex and tries to memorize the training data instead of learning the underlying patterns. It's like a student who memorizes answers without understanding the concepts in a textbook. Consider a spam email filter. If we train a model on a dataset of spam and non-spam emails, an overly complex model might remember each email's unique characteristics, including typos, font styles, or specific keywords. As a result, it would struggle to generalize to new, unseen emails, marking some legitimate ones as spam and vice versa.

Machine learning aims to find the right level of model complexity, a balance between underfitting and overfitting. This sweet spot is where the model generalizes well to new, unseen data. Achieving this balance requires careful model selection, feature engineering, and tuning. Let's explore how to identify and address both underfitting and overfitting.

Signs of underfitting can be:

- High training error (i.e., model performs poorly even on the training data).

- High validation error (i.e., model performs poorly on new data).

- The model's predictions are too simplistic and inaccurate.

The possible solutions can be:

- Increase model complexity: Choose a more complex algorithm or increase the model's capacity (e.g., using a deeper neural network).

- Add relevant features: Incorporate more meaningful features from the data to help the model learn better.

Signs of overfitting can be:

- Low training error (i.e., model fits the training data almost perfectly).

- High validation error (i.e., model performs poorly on new data).

- The model's predictions are overly sensitive to noise in the training data.

Solutions for overfitting can be:

- *Reduce model complexity*: Simplify the model architecture by reducing the number of features, nodes in a neural network, or tree depth in decision trees.

- Strengthen regularization techniques.

- *Get more data*: Additional high-quality data can help the model generalize better.

- Employ techniques like k-fold cross-validation to evaluate model performance more robustly.

Let's apply these concepts to a real-world problem: image classification. Suppose we want to build a machine-learning model that can distinguish between cats and dogs based on images. If we use a simple algorithm, like logistic regression, to classify these images, it might need help to capture the intricate details that differentiate cats from dogs, resulting in poor accuracy. That is the underfitting scenario.

Conversely, suppose we employ an intense neural network with millions of parameters and train it on a relatively small dataset. In that case, the model may memorize the training images' pixel values rather than learning meaningful features. This leads to high training accuracy but needs to improve generalization to new, unseen cat and dog images. That is overfitting scenario.

1.7.2 Other Limitations

The efficacy of machine learning models heavily hinges on the quality and quantity of data. Noisy or biased data can result in inaccurate predictions. Furthermore, obtaining labeled data for supervised learning can be costly and time-consuming. Machine learning models can inherit biases from the training data, culminating in unfair or discriminatory outcomes. Ensuring fairness and mitigating bias in models stands as a critical ethical concern. Deep learning models, in particular, often assume the guise of "black boxes" due to the intricacy of understanding their decision-making processes. Interpretability is crucial, especially in high-stakes domains such as healthcare and finance. Machine learning's heavy reliance on data is fundamental. Data quality and quantity significantly affect algorithm performance. Biased, incomplete, or unrepresentative data can lead to accurate or fair predictions. Collecting and labeling large datasets can be time-consuming and costly, posing challenges for specific applications.

Machine learning models often need help to generalize beyond their training data. While they may excel in the training data, they can fail on unseen or out-of-distribution data, known as overfitting. Overfitting occurs when models become too specialized in capturing noise in the training data, hampering generalization. Addressing overfitting requires model selection, regularization, and cross-validation. Many machine learning models, intense learning models, are viewed as black boxes. They provide predictions, but understanding why a particular decision was made can be challenging. This lack of interpretability and explainability is problematic in critical domains like healthcare or finance, where trust and accountability require understanding the model's reasoning. Machine learning models can unintentionally perpetuate biases from the training data. Biases related to race, gender, or other sensitive attributes in the training data may lead to biased predictions. Mitigating bias and ensuring fairness is an ongoing challenge, requiring careful data preprocessing, algorithmic fairness techniques, and ongoing monitoring. Some shot notes of related problems can be described below.

- Machine learning models, especially those in recommendation systems and personalized advertising, rely on user data, raising significant privacy concerns. Mishandling sensitive data can lead to privacy breaches and personal information leaks. Balancing model utility with user privacy is an ongoing challenge.

- Many machine learning models, intense learning models, demand substantial computational resources. This includes high-performance hardware and energy consumption, making them inaccessible to smaller organizations and raising environmental concerns. Efficient model architectures and optimization techniques are developed to address these resource limitations.

- Machine learning models excel at finding correlations but struggle with causality. While they predict outcomes based on data patterns, they cannot establish underlying cause-and-effect relationships. This limitation is crucial in domains where causality is essential, such as scientific research and public policy.

- Machine learning models assume data distributions remain constant over time. However, real-world data distributions can change due to various factors, leading to concept drift. Models that do not adapt to these changes may become obsolete, necessitating continuous monitoring and retraining.

- Machine learning models lack the common sense and contextual understanding humans naturally possess. While they may make data-driven predictions, they lack the intuition and contextual knowledge humans use for decision-making. This limitation hinders their suitability for tasks requiring a deep understanding of the world.

1.8 CONCLUSION

Smart assisted homes and machine learning are two technological innovations fundamentally changing how we experience our living environments. A smart assisted home, commonly known as a smart home, incorporates interconnected devices and systems that can be managed and automated through technology. Machine learning, a subset of AI, empowers these smart homes by allowing them to learn from data and make informed decisions without explicit programming. The application of machine learning within smart homes is reshaping home automation. Machine learning algorithms can analyze data from various sensors and devices in the home, including motion sensors, temperature detectors, and cameras. They then use this data to understand and predict patterns of user behavior. For example, a smart home system can learn when occupants usually return home from work and adjust lighting, temperature, and security accordingly. Over time, these systems become more attuned to the inhabitants' routines, making the home more comfortable and efficient. Energy management is another critical area where machine learning is making a significant impact in smart homes. By utilizing historical data and real-time environmental conditions, machine learning algorithms can optimize the operation of heating, cooling, and lighting systems. A smart thermostat equipped with machine learning can adapt heating and cooling schedules to minimize energy consumption while maintaining comfort levels. This not only reduces energy costs but also contributes to environmental sustainability. Security and safety are paramount concerns in any household, and machine learning is crucial in enhancing these aspects within smart homes. Machine learning also contributes significantly to improving the user experience in smart homes. Natural language processing (NLP) algorithms enable voice assistants like Amazon's Alexa and

Google Assistant to comprehend and respond to spoken commands. These voice-activated assistants can control various smart devices, provide answers to questions, and offer information, making it more convenient for homeowners to interact with their homes. Health and well-being increasingly become focal points for smart homes, and machine learning enhances these aspects. Wearable devices and health sensors can gather data on an individual's vital signs and daily activities. Machine learning algorithms can analyze this data to offer personalized health recommendations and identify anomalies that may indicate health issues. For example, a smart home system can alert caregivers or medical professionals if it detects a sudden change in an older adult's mobility patterns or vital signs. Furthermore, machine learning facilitates predictive maintenance for smart home devices. By examining data from appliances and systems, it can predict when a device is likely to require maintenance or face potential failure. Homeowners can receive proactive notifications and schedule repairs or replacements before a breakdown occurs, ensuring uninterrupted functionality in their smart homes. In conclusion, the incorporation of machine learning into smart assisted homes is revolutionizing the way we interact with and manage our living spaces. From automation and energy efficiency to security, convenience, and health monitoring, machine learning algorithms enhance every facet of smart homes. As these technologies advance, smart homes will become even more intuitive and adaptive, providing homeowners with heightened comfort and control while promoting a more sustainable and secure future.

REFERENCES

[1] L. Heron, "Smart Solutions for Seniors [Smart Homes - Consumer Technology]," *Engineering & Technology*, vol. 18, no. 3, pp. 42–45, 2023, doi: 10.1049/et.2023.0308

[2] (a) A. Friedman, "Homes for Changing Times," *The Urban Book Series*, pp. 1–29, 2023, doi: 10.1007/978-3-031-35368-0_1. (b) C. Warner Frieson, "Predictors of Recurrent Falls in Community-Dwelling Older Adults after Fall-Related Hip Fracture," *Journal of Perioperative & Critical Intensive Care Nursing*, vol. 2, no. 2, pp. 1–2, 2016.

[3] L. Vijayaraja, N. S. Jayakumar, R. Dhanasekar, M. P. Manibha, V. Vignesh, and R. Kesavan, "Sustainable Smart Homes Using IoT for Future Smart Cities," in: *2023 4th International Conference on Smart Electronics and Communication (ICOSEC)*, Tamil Nadu, India, Sep 20-22, 2023, doi: 10.1109/icosec58147.2023.10276371

[4] M. A. Fiatarone Singh, "Exercise, Nutrition and Managing Hip Fracture in Older Persons," *Current Opinion in Clinical Nutrition and Metabolic Care*, vol. 1, no. 1, p. 1, Nov 2013.

[5] M. Alwan, S. Dalal, D. Mack, S. Kell, B. Turner, J. Leachtenauer, and R. Felder, "Impact of Monitoring Technology in Assisted Living: Outcome Pilot," *IEEE Transactions on Information Technology in Biomedicine*, vol. 10, no. 1, pp. 192–198, Jan 2006.

[6] C. N. Scanaill, S. Carew, P. Barralon, N. Noury, D. Lyons, and G. M. Lyons, "A Review of Approaches to Mobility Telemonitoring of the Elderly in Their Living Environment," *Annals of Biomedical Engineering*, vol. 34, no. 4, pp. 547–563, Mar 2006.

[7] M. Perry, A. Dowdall, L. Lines, and K. Hone, "Multimodal and Ubiquitous Computing Systems: Supporting Independent-living Older Users," in: *IEEE Transactions on Information Technology in Biomedicine*, vol. 8, no. 3, pp. 258–270, Sep 2004.

[8] R. Al-Shaqi, M. Mourshed, and Y. Rezgui, "Progress in Ambient Assisted Systems for Independent Living by the Elderly," *SpringerPlus*, vol. 5, no. 1, May 2016, doi: doi.org/10.1186/s40064-016-2272-8

[9] Q. Ni, A. García Hernando, and I. de la Cruz, "The Elderly's Independent Living in Smart Homes: A Characterization of Activities and Sensing Infrastructure Survey to Facilitate Services Development," *Sensors*, vol. 15, no. 5, pp. 11312–11362, May 2015.

[10] M. R. Alam, M. B. I. Reaz, and M. A. M. Ali, "A Review of Smart Homes—Past, Present, and Future," in: *IEEE Transactions on Systems, Man, and Cybernetics, Part C (Applications and Reviews)*, vol. 42, no. 6, pp. 1190–1203, Nov 2012.

[11] P. Rashidi and A. Mihailidis, "A Survey on Ambient-Assisted Living Tools for Older Adults," *IEEE Journal of Biomedical and Health Informatics*, vol. 17, no. 3, pp. 579–590, May 2013.

[12] A. S. M. Salih and A. Abraham, "A Review of Ambient Intelligence Assisted Healthcare Monitoring," *International Journal of Computer Information Systems and Industrial Management Applications*, vol. 5, pp. 741–750, 2013.

[13] K. K. B. Peetoom, M. A. S. Lexis, M. Joore, C. D. Dirksen, and L. P. De Witte, "Literature Review on Monitoring Technologies and Their Outcomes in Independently Living Elderly People," *Disability and Rehabilitation: Assistive Technology*, vol. 10, no. 4, pp. 271–294, Sep 2014.

[14] R. Khusainov, D. Azzi, I. Achumba, and S. Bersch, "Real-Time Human Ambulation, Activity, and Physiological Monitoring: Taxonomy of Issues, Techniques, Applications, Challenges and Limitations," *Sensors*, vol. 13, no. 10, pp. 12852–12902, Sep 2013.

[15] A. Avci, S. Bosch, M. Marin-Perianu, R. Marin-Perianu, and P. Havinga, "Activity Recognition Using Inertial Sensing for Healthcare, Wellbeing and Sports Applications: A Survey," in: *23rd International Conference on Architecture of Computing Systems*, Hannover, Germany, pp. 1–10, 2010.

[16] A. Bulling, U. Blanke, and B. Schiele, "A Tutorial on Human Activity Recognition Using Body-worn Inertial Sensors," *ACM Computing Surveys*, vol. 46, no. 3, pp. 1–33, Jan 2014.

[17] S. Helal, W. Mann, H. El-Zabadani, J. King, Y. Kaddoura, and E. Jansen, "The Gator Tech Smart House: A Programmable Pervasive Space," *Computer*, vol. 38, no. 3, pp. 50–60, Mar 2005.

[18] J. Cook, A. S. Crandall, B. L. Thomas, and N. C. Krishnan, "CASAS: A Smart Home in a Box," *Computer*, vol. 46, no. 7, pp. 62–69, Jul 2013.

[19] M. Vacher, B. Lecouteux, P. Chahuara, F. Portet, B. Meillon, and N. Bonnefond, "The Sweet-Home Speech and Multimodal Corpus for Home Automation Interaction," in: *Proceedings of the Ninth International Conference on Language Resources and Evaluation (LREC'14)*, Reykjavik, Iceland, pp. 4499–4506, 2014.

[20] J. Lloret, A. Canovas, S. Sendra, and L. Parra, "A Smart Communication Architecture for Ambient Assisted Living," in *IEEE Communications Magazine*, vol. 53, no. 1, pp. 26–33, Jan 2015, doi: 10.1109/MCOM.2015.7010512

[21] B. Andó, S. Baglio, C. O. Lombardo, and V. Marletta, A Multisensor Data-Fusion Approach for ADL and Fall Classification. *IEEE Transactions on Instrumentation and Measurement*, vol. 65, pp. 1960–1967, 2016.

[22] S. Badgujar and A. S. Pillai, "Fall Detection for Elderly People using Machine Learning," in: *Proceedings of the 11th International Conference on Computing, Communication and Networking Technologies (ICCCNT)*, Kharagpur, India, Jul 1–3, 2020.

[23] J. Xie, K. Guo, Z. Zhou, Y. Yan, and P. Yang, "ART: Adaptive and Real-time Fall Detection Using COTS Smart Watch," in: *Proceedings of the 6th International Conference on Big Data Computing and Communications (BIGCOM)*, Deqing, China, Jul 24–25, 2020.

[24] M. Nouredanesh, K. Gordt, M. Schwenk, and J. Tung Automated Detection of Multidirectional Compensatory Balance Reactions: A Step Towards Tracking Naturally Occurring Near Falls, *IEEE Transactions on Neural Systems and Rehabilitation Engineering*, vol. 28, pp. 478–487, 2020.

[25] D. Sarabia, R. Usach, C. Palau, and M. Esteve, "Highly-Efficient Fog-Based Deep Learning Aal Fall Detection System," *Internet Things*, vol. 11, p. 100185, 2020.

[26] R. Z. Ur Rehman, C. Buckley, M. E. Micó-Amigo, C. Kirk, M. Dunne-Willows, C. Mazzá, J. Qing Shi, L. Alcock, L. Rochester, and S. Del Din, "Accelerometry-Based Digital Gait Characteristics

for Classification of Parkinson's Disease: What Counts?," *IEEE Open Journal of Engineering in Medicine and Biology*, vol. 1, pp. 65–73, 2020 [CrossRef].

[27] R. Lutze, "Practicality of Smartwatch Apps for Supporting Elderly People—A Comprehensive Survey," in: *Proceedings of the IEEE International Conference on Engineering, Technology and Innovation (ICE/ITMC)*, Stuttgart, Germany, pp. 17–20 Jun 2018.

[28] B. Andó, S. Baglio, C. O. Lombardo, and V. Marletta, "An Event Polarized Paradigm for ADL Detection in AAL Context," *IEEE Transactions on Instrumentation and Measurement*, vol. 64, pp. 1814–1825, 2015 [CrossRef].

[29] M. Haghi, A. Geissler, H. Fleischer, N. Stoll, and K. Thurow, "Ubiqsense: A Personal Wearable in Ambient Parameters Monitoring based on IoT Platform," in: *Proceedings of the International Conference on Sensing and Instrumentation in IoT Era (ISSI)*, Lisbon, Portugal, Aug 29–30, 2019.

[30] L. Scalise, V. Petrini, V. Di Mattia, P. Russo, A. De Leo, G. Manfredi, and G. Cerri, "Multiparameter Electromagnetic Sensor for AAL Indoor Measurement of the Respiration Rate and Position of a Subject," in: *Proceedings of the IEEE International Instrumentation and Measurement Technology Conference (I2MTC)*, Pisa, Italy, May 11–14, 2015.

[31] A. L. Bleda-Tomas, R. Maestre-Ferriz, M. Á. Beteta-Medina, and J. A. Vidal-Poveda, "AmICare: Ambient Intelligent and Assistive System for Caregivers support," in: *Proceedings of the IEEE 16th International Conference on Embedded and Ubiquitous Computing (EUC)*, Bucharest, Romania, Oct 29–31, 2018.

[32] M. P. Fanti, G. Faraut, J. J. Lesage, and M. Roccotelli, "An Integrated Framework for Binary Sensor Placement and Inhabitants Location Tracking," *IEEE Transactions on Systems, Man, and Cybernetics*, vol. 48, pp. 154–160, 2018 [CrossRef].

[33] P. De, A. Chatterjee, and A. Rakshit, "PIR Sensor based AAL Tool for Human Movement Detection: Modified MCP based Dictionary Learning Approach," *IEEE Transactions on Instrumentation and Measurement*, vol. 69, pp. 7377–7385, 2020 [CrossRef].

[34] A. R. Jimenez, F. Seco, P. Peltola, and M. Espinilla, "Location of Persons Using Binary Sensors and BLE Beacons for Ambient Assistive Living," in: *Proceedings of the 2018 International Conference on Indoor Positioning and Indoor Navigation (IPIN)*, Nantes, France, Sep 24–27, 2018.

[35] C. Guerra, V. Bianchi, I. De Munari, and P. Ciampolini, "CARDEAGate: Low-cost, ZigBee-based Localization and Identification for AAL Purposes," in: *Proceedings of the IEEE International Instrumentation and Measurement Technology Conference (I2MTC) Proceedings*, Pisa, Italy, May 11–14, 2015.

[36] S. Chen, "Toward Ambient Assistance: A Spatially Aware Virtual Assistant eNabled by Object Detection," in: *Proceedings of the International Conference on Computer Engineering and Application (ICCEA)*, Guangzhou, China, Mar 18–20, 2020.

[37] S. Yue, Y. Yang, H. Wang, H. Rahul, and D. Katabi, "BodyCompass: Monitoring Sleep Posture with Wireless Signals," *Proceedings of the ACM on Interactive, Mobile, Wearable and Ubiquitous Technologies*, vol. 4, pp. 1–25, 2020 [CrossRef].

[38] L. Fan, T. Li, Y. Yuan, and D. Katabi, "In-Home Daily-Life Captioning Using Radio Signals. Computer Science—ECCV," *arXiv*, 2020, arXiv:2008.10966.

[39] V. Vahia, Z. Kabelac, C. YuHsu, B. Forester, P. Monette, R. May, K. Hobbs, U. Munir, K. Hoti, and D. Katabi, "Radio Signal Sensing and Signal Processing to Monitor Behavioural Symptoms in Dementia: A Case Study,". *The American Journal of Geriatric Psychiatry*, vol. 28, pp. 820–825, 2020 [CrossRef] [PubMed].

[40] L. Li, Y. Shuang, Q. Ma, H. Li, H. Zhao, M. L. Wei, C. Liu, C. Hao, C. Qiu, and T. Cui, "Intelligent Metasurface Imager and Recognizer," *Light: Science & Applications*, vol. 8, p. 97, 2019 [CrossRef].

[41] P. del Hougne M. Imani, A. Diebold, R. Horstmeyer, and D. Smith, "Learned Integrated Sensing Pipeline: Reconfigurable Metasurface Transceivers as Trainable Physical Layer in an Artificial Neural Network," *Advanced Science*, vol. 7, p. 1901913, 2020 [CrossRef].

[42] H. Y. Li, H. T. Zhao, M. L. Wei, H. X. Ruan, Y. Shuang, T. J. Cui, P. del Hougne, and L. Li, "Intelligent Electromagnetic Sensing with Learnable Data Acquisition and Processing," *Patterns*, vol. 1, p. 100006, 2020 [CrossRef].

[43] I. Cebanov, C. Dobre, A. Gradinar, R. I. Ciobanu, and V. D. Stanciu, "Activity Recognition for Ambient Assisted Living Using off-the Shelf Motion Sensing Input Devices," in: *Proceedings of the Global IoT Summit (GIoTS)*, Aarhus, Denmark, Jun 17–21, 2019.

[44] K. Ryselis, T. Petkus, T. Blazauskas, R. Maskeliunas, and R. Damasevicius, "Multiple Kinect Based System to Monitor and Analyze Key Performance Indicators of Physical Training," *Human-centric Computing and Information Sciences*, vol. 10, p. 51, 2020 [CrossRef].

[45] D. Austin, T. L. Hayes, J. Kaye, N. Mattek, and M. Pavel, "On the Disambiguation of Passively Measured In-home Gait Velocities from Multi-person Smart Homes", *Journal of Ambient Intelligence and Smart Environments*, vol. 3, no. 2, pp. 165–174, Apr. 2011.

[46] D. Austin, T. L. Hayes, J. Kaye, N. Mattek, and M. Pavel, "Unobtrusive Monitoring of the Longitudinal Evolution of In-home Gait Velocity Data with Applications to Elder Care," in: *2011 Annual International Conference of the IEEE Engineering in Medicine and Biology Society*, pp. 6495–6498, Aug 2011.

[47] T. S. Barger, D. E. Brown, and M. Alwan, "Health-Status Monitoring Through Analysis of Behavioural Patterns," *IEEE Transactions on Systems, Man, and Cybernetics - Part A: Systems and Humans*, vol. 35, no. 1, pp. 22–27, Jan 2005.

[48] B. G. Celler, W. Earnshaw, E. D. Ilsar, L. Betbeder-Matibet, M. F. Harris, R. Clark, T. Hesketh, and N. H. Lovell, "Remote Monitoring of Health Status of the Elderly at Home. A Multidisciplinary Project on Aging at the University of New South Wales," *International Journal of Bio-Medical Computing*, vol. 40, no. 2, pp. 147–155, Oct 1995.

[49] D. J. Cook and M. Schmitter-Edgecombe, "Assessing the Quality of Activities in a Smart Environment," *Methods of Information in Medicine*, vol. 48, no. 5, pp. 480–485, May 2009.

[50] S. Dalai, M. Alwan, R. Seifrafi, S. Kell, and D. Brown, "A Rule-Based Approach to the Analysis of Elders' Activity Data: Detection of Health and Possible Emergency Conditions", in: *AAAI Fall 2005 Symposium (EMBC)*, Sep 2005.

[51] J. Demongeot, G. Virone, F. Duchêne, G. Benchetrit, T. Hervé, N. Noury, and V. Rialle, "Multi-sensors Acquisition, Data Fusion, Knowledge Mining and Alarm Triggering in Health Smart Homes for Elderly People," *Comptes Rendus Biologies*, vol. 325, no. 6, pp. 673–682, Jun 2002.

[52] F. J. Fernández-Luque, J. Zapata, and R. Ruiz, "A System for Ubiquitous Fall Monitoring at Home Via a Wireless Sensor Network," in: *Annual International Conference of the IEEE Engineering in Medicine and Biology*, pp. 2246–2249, Aug 2010.

[53] C. Franco, J. Demongeot, C. Villemazet, and N. Vuillerme, "Behavioural Telemonitoring of the Elderly at Home: Detection of Nycthemeral Rhythms Drifts from Location Data," in *IEEE 24th International Conference on Advanced Information Networking and Applications Workshops*, pp. 759–766, 2010.

[54] A. Glascock and D. Kutzik, "The Impact of Behavioural Monitoring Technology on the Provision of Health Care in the Home," *Journal of Universal Computer Science*, vol. 12, no. 1, pp. 59–79, 2006.

[55] A. P. Glascock and D. M. Kutzik, "Behavioural Telemedicine: A New Approach to the Continuous Nonintrusive Monitoring of Activities of Daily Living," *Telemedicine Journal*, vol. 6, no. 1, pp. 33–44, May 2000.

[56] S. Hagler, D. Austin, T. L. Hayes, J. Kaye, and M. Pavel, "Unobtrusive and Ubiquitous In-Home Monitoring: A Methodology for Continuous Assessment of Gait Velocity in Elders," *IEEE Transactions on Biomedical Engineering*, vol. 57, no. 4, pp. 813–820, Apr 2010.

[57] T. L. Hayes, M. Pavel, and J. A. Kaye, "An Unobtrusive In-home Monitoring System for Detection of Key Motor Changes Preceding Cognitive Decline," in: *The 26th Annual International Conference of the IEEE Engineering in Medicine and Biology Society*, pp. 2480–2483, 2004.

[58] J. Johnson, *Consumer Response to Home Monitoring: A Survey of Older Consumers and Informal Care Providers*, Florida: University of Florida, 2009.

[59] A. R. Kaushik, N. H. Lovell, and B. G. Celler, "Evaluation of PIR Detector Characteristics for Monitoring Occupancy Patterns of Elderly People Living Alone at Home," in: *29th Annual International Conference of the IEEE Engineering in Medicine and Biology Society*, pp. 3802–3805, Aug 2007.

[60] J. Kaye, "Intelligent Systems for Assessment of Aging Changes (ISAAC): Deploying Unobtrusive Home-based Technology," *Gerontechnology*, vol. 9, no. 2, Apr 2010.

[61] M. Abidine and B. Fergani, "News Schemes for Activity Recognition Systems Using PCA-WSVM, ICA-WSVM, and LDA-WSVM," *Information*, vol. 6, no. 3, pp. 505–521, Aug 2015.

[62] J. Aertssen, M. Rudinac, and P. Jonker, *Fall and Action Detection in Elderly Homes*, Maastricht, The Netherlands: AAATE, 2011.

[63] E. Auvinet, L. Reveret, A. St-Arnaud, J. Rousseau, and J. Meunier, "Fall Detection Using Multiple Cameras," in *30th Annual International Conference of the IEEE Engineering in Medicine and Biology Society*, Vancouver, BC, pp. 2554–2557, 2008.

[64] E. Auvinet, F. Multon, A. Saint-Arnaud, J. Rousseau, and J. Meunier, "Fall Detection With Multiple Cameras: An Occlusion-Resistant Method Based on 3-D Silhouette Vertical Distribution," *IEEE Transactions on Information Technology in Biomedicine*, vol. 15, no. 2, pp. 290–300, Mar 2011.

[65] M. Belshaw, B. Taati, D. Giesbrecht, and A. Mihailidis, "Intelligent Vision-based Fall Detection System: Preliminary Results from a Realworld Deployment," in: *Rehabilitation Engineering and Assistive Technology Society of North America (RESNA)*, pp. 1–4, 2011.

[66] M. Belshaw, B. Taati, J. Snoek, and A. Mihailidis, "Towards a Single Sensor Passive Solution for Automated Fall Detection," in: *Proceedings of the 33rd Annual International Conference of the IEEE EMBS*, pp. 1773–1776, Aug/Sep 2011.

[67] S. J. Berlin and M. John, "Human Interaction Recognition Through Deep Learning Network," in: *IEEE International Carnahan Conference on Security Technology (ICCST)*, Orlando, FL, pp. 1–4, 2016.

[68] D. Brulin, Y. Benezeth, and E. Courtial, "Posture Recognition Based on Fuzzy Logic for Home Monitoring of the Elderly," in *IEEE Transactions on Information Technology in Biomedicine*, vol. 16, no. 5, pp. 974–982, Sep. 2012.

[69] H. Chen, G. Wang, J. H. Xue, and L. He, "A Novel Hierarchical Framework for Human Action Recognition," *Pattern Recognition*, vol. 55, pp. 148–159, 2016.

[70] C. W. Lin and Z. H. Ling, "Automatic Fall Incident Detection in Compressed Video for Intelligent Homecare," in: *2007 16th International Conference on Computer Communications and Networks*, Honolulu, HI, pp. 1172–1177, 2007.

[71] Y. Du, W. Wang, and L. Wang, "Hierarchical Recurrent Neural Network for Skeleton Based Action Recognition," in: *IEEE Conference on Computer Vision and Pattern Recognition (CVPR)*, pp. 1110–1118, Boston, MA, 2015.

[72] H. Foroughi, B. S. Aski, and H. Pourreza, "Intelligent Video Surveillance for Monitoring Fall Detection of Elderly in Home Environments," in: *11th International Conference on Computer and Information Technology*, Khulna, pp. 219–224, 2008.

[73] Z. Huang, C. Wan, T. Probst, and L. V. Gool, *Deep Learning on lie Groups for Skeleton-Based Action Recognition, arXiv Prepr*, Cornell University Library, Ithaca, NY, 2016, http://arxiv.org/abs/1612.05877

[74] M. Kreković et al., "A Method for Real-time Detection of Human Fall from Video," in: *Proceedings of the 35th International Convention MIPRO*, Opatija, pp. 1709–1712, 2012.

[75] Z. Lan, M. Lin, X. Li, A. G. Hauptmann, and B. Raj, "Beyond Gaussian Pyramid: Multi-skip Feature Stacking for Action Recognition," in: *IEEE Conference on Computer Vision and Pattern Recognition (CVPR)*, pp. 204–212, Boston, MA, 2015.

[76] Y. Li, W. Li, V. Mahadevan, and N. Vasconcelos, "Vlad3: Encoding Dynamics of Deep Features for Action Recognition," in: *IEEE Conference on Computer Vision and Pattern Recognition (CVPR)*, pp. 1951–1960, Las Vegas, NV, 2016.

[77] Y. Li, K. C. Ho, and M. Popescu, "A Microphone Array System for Automatic Fall Detection," *IEEE Transactions on Biomedical Engineering*, vol. 59, no. 5, pp. 1291–1301, May 2012.

[78] Y. Lee, J. Kim, M. Son, and M. Lee, "Implementation of Accelerometer Sensor Module and Fall Detection Monitoring System based on Wireless Sensor Network," in: *29th Annual International Conference of the IEEE Engineering in Medicine and Biology Society*, Lyon, pp. 2315–2318, 2007.

[79] T. Lee and A. Mihailidis, "An Intelligent Emergency Response System: Preliminary Development and Testing of Automated Fall Detection," *Journal of Telemedicine and Telecare*, vol. 11, no. 4, pp. 194–198, 2005.

[80] Y.-S. Lee and W.-Y. Chung, "Visual Sensor Based Abnormal Event Detection with Moving Shadow Removal in Home Healthcare Applications," *Sensors*, vol. 12, no. 12, pp. 573–584, Jan 2012.

[81] J. Lien, N. Gillian, M. E. Karagozler, P. Amihood, C. Schwesig, E. Olson, H. Raja, and I. Poupyrev, "Soli," *ACM Transactions on Graphics*, vol. 35, no. 4, pp. 1–19, Jul 2016.

[82] L. Rui, S. Chen, K. C. Ho, M. Rantz, and M. Skubic, "Estimation of Human Walking Speed by Doppler Radar for Elderly Care," *Journal of Ambient Intelligence and Smart Environments*, vol. 9, no. 2, pp. 181–191, Feb 2017.

[83] Q. Wan, Y. Li, C. Li, and R. Pal, "Gesture Recognition for Smart Home Applications Using Portable Radar Sensors," in: *36th Annual International Conference of the IEEE Engineering in Medicine and Biology Society*, Chicago, IL, pp. 6414–6417, 2014.

[84] F. Thullier, A. Beaulieu, J. Maître, S. Gaboury, and K. Bouchard, "A Systematic Evaluation of the XeThru X4 Ultra-Wideband Radar Behaviour," *Procedia Computer Science*, vol. 198, pp. 148–155, 2022.

[85] M. Z. Uddin, F. M. Noori, and J. Torresen, "In-Home Emergency Detection Using an Ambient Ultra-Wideband Radar Sensor and Deep Learning," 2020 *IEEE Ukrainian Microwave Week (UkrMW)*, 2020, pp. 1089–1093, doi: 10.1109/UkrMW49653.2020.9252708

[86] F. M. Noori, M. Z. Uddin, and J. Torresen, "Ultra-Wideband Radar-Based Activity Recognition Using Deep Learning," in *IEEE Access*, vol. 9, pp. 138132–138143, 2021, doi: 10.1109/ACCESS.2021.3117667

[87] H. Xu, M. P. Ebrahim, K. Hasan, F. Heydari, P. Howley, and M. R. Yuce, "Accurate Heart Rate and Respiration Rate Detection Based on a Higher-Order Harmonics Peak Selection Method Using Radar Non-Contact Sensors," *Sensors*, vol. 22, p. 83, 2022.

[88] S. Klavestad, G. Assres, S. Fagernes, and T.-M. Grønli, "Monitoring Activities of Daily Living Using UWB Radar Technology: A Contactless Approach," *IoT*, vol. 1, pp. 320–336, 2020.

[89] M. Liu, "Machine Learning: An Overview," *Machine Learning, Animated*, Chapman and Hall/CRC, pp. 34–46, Oct. 2023, doi: 10.1201/b23383-3

[90] D. Chopra and R. Khurana, "Introduction To Machine Learning," *Introduction to Machine Learning with Python, Bentham Science Publishers*, pp. 15–29, Feb 2023, doi: 10.2174/97898151 24422123010004

[91] M. Plaue, "Supervised Machine Learning," *Data Science*, pp. 185–248, 2023, doi: 10.1007/978-3-662-67882-4_6

[92] H. Li, "Summary of Supervised Learning Methods," *Machine Learning Methods*, pp. 273–280, Dec 2023, doi: 10.1007/978-981-99-3917-6_12

[93] T. Jo, "Unsupervised Learning," *Deep Learning Foundations*, pp. 57–81, 2023, doi: 10.1007/978-3-031-32879-4_3

[94] H. Li, "Introduction to Unsupervised Learning," *Machine Learning Methods*, pp. 281–292, Dec 2023, doi: 10.1007/978-981-99-3917-6_13

[95] J. Kim, S. Park, S.-D. Roh, and K.-S. Chung, "An Efficient Noisy Label Learning Method with Semi-supervised Learning," in: *Proceedings of the 2023 6th International Conference on Machine Vision and Applications*, March 2023, doi: 10.1145/3589572.3589596

[96] J. Saeedi and A. Giusti, "Semi-supervised Visual Anomaly Detection Based on Convolutional Autoencoder and Transfer Learning," *Machine Learning with Applications*, vol. 11, p. 100451, Mar 2023, doi: 10.1016/j.mlwa.2023.100451

[97] Z. Şen, "Deep Learning," *Shallow and Deep Learning Principles*, pp. 621–658, 2023, doi: 10.1007/978-3-031-29555-3_9

[98] J. Wang, "Instance-based Transfer Learning," *Introduction to Transfer Learning*, 2023, doi: 10.1007/978-981-99-1109-7_2

[99] P. Sarang, "Transfer Learning," *Mastering the Modern Data Science Process*, 2023, doi: 10.1007/978-3-031-39601-4_7

[100] M. Rostami, H. He, M. Chen, and D. Roth, "Transfer Learning via Representation Learning," *Adaptation, Learning, and Optimization*, pp. 233–257, Oct 2022, doi: 10.1007/978-3-031-11748-0_10

## CHAPTER 2

Python and Its Libraries

2.1 PYTHON'S KEY FEATURES

Python, a dynamic and high-level programming language, stands out for its readability and simplicity, designed by Guido van Rossum. Its syntax allows developers to express concepts in fewer lines of code than languages like C++ or Java, making it beginner-friendly. Python's versatility is evident in its applications, from web development to data science and artificial intelligence [1–10]. The language's strength lies in its extensive standard libraries, fostering rapid development. Its open-source nature and supportive community contribute to its popularity. Python's readability and powerful capabilities make it a preferred choice for a broad spectrum of programming tasks in today's tech landscape.

Python's popularity can be attributed to its numerous features, which make it an excellent choice for both beginners and professionals:

- Python's syntax is straightforward to understand, making it an ideal language for those new to programming. Using indentation for code blocks enforces a consistent and clean coding style.

- It is a versatile language that can be used for various applications, from web development to scientific computing, data analysis, and artificial intelligence. This versatility has contributed to its widespread adoption across industries.

- It boasts an extensive standard library that covers a wide range of functionality, making it easy to perform everyday tasks without needing third-party libraries. Additionally, there is a vast ecosystem of third-party libraries and frameworks that extend Python's capabilities further.

- It is available on various platforms, including Windows, macOS, and Linux. This cross-platform compatibility ensures that Python code can be written and executed on different operating systems without significant modifications.

DOI: 10.1201/9781003425908-2

- It has a large and active community of developers who contribute to its growth and provide support through forums, mailing lists, and social media. This strong community support ensures that a wealth of resources is available for Python learners and professionals alike.

- It is an open-source language, meaning its source code is freely available for anyone to view, modify, and distribute. This open nature has fostered collaboration and innovation within the Python community.

2.2 PYTHON IN PRACTICE

Python's versatility and simplicity have led to its widespread adoption in various fields. Let's explore some of the critical applications of Python:

- Python has a thriving ecosystem of web development frameworks, including Django, Flask, and Pyramid. These frameworks simplify the process of building web applications, making Python a popular choice for web developers. Django, in particular, is known for its robustness and follows the "batteries-included" philosophy, providing a wide range of built-in tools and libraries.

- It is a powerhouse for data analysis and visualization. Libraries like NumPy, pandas, and Matplotlib make it easy to work with data, perform statistical analysis, and create compelling visualizations. Data scientists and analysts often use Jupyter Notebooks to interactively explore data and share their findings.

- It is the go-to language for machine learning and artificial intelligence (AI) projects. Libraries like TensorFlow, PyTorch, and scikit-learn provide powerful tools for developing and training machine learning models. Python's simplicity and extensive libraries have made it accessible to researchers and developers in the AI field.

- Scientists and researchers across various disciplines use Python for scientific computing. Libraries like SciPy, SymPy, and AstroML offer specialized tools for numerical optimization, symbolic mathematics, and astronomy data analysis.

- Python's ease of use makes it an excellent choice for automation and scripting tasks. System administrators, for example, rely on Python scripts to automate repetitive tasks, manage servers, and perform system maintenance.

- Python is also used in IoT projects due to its versatility and support for various hardware platforms. Raspberry Pi, a popular single-board computer for IoT projects, supports Python, making it a preferred language for building IoT applications.

- NLP is a subfield of AI that focuses on the interaction between computers and human language. Python's NLTK (Natural Language Toolkit) and spaCy libraries are commonly used for NLP tasks like text classification, sentiment analysis, and language modeling.

2.3 PYTHON LIBRARIES AND FRAMEWORKS

Python's strength lies in its core language features and its extensive ecosystem of libraries and frameworks. These libraries simplify complex tasks, accelerate development, and enable developers to build robust applications more efficiently. Here are some of the most prominent Python libraries and frameworks.

NumPy is a fundamental library for numerical computing in Python. It supports large, multi-dimensional arrays and matrices and various high-level mathematical functions to operate on these arrays. NumPy is a foundational library for data science and scientific computing.

Pandas is a data manipulation and analysis library that simplifies working with structured data. It introduces data structures like DataFrames and Series, which are essential for tasks such as data cleaning, exploration, and transformation.

Matplotlib is a popular library for creating static, animated, or interactive visualizations in Python. It offers various plotting functions and styles, making it suitable for data scientists, researchers, and engineers.

Scikit-learn is a machine-learning library that provides tools for classification, regression, clustering, dimensionality reduction, and more. It is widely used in academia and industry for developing and deploying machine learning models.

TensorFlow and PyTorch are deep learning frameworks that have revolutionized the field of artificial intelligence. They allow developers to build and train neural networks for tasks like image recognition, natural language processing, and reinforcement learning.

These are just a few examples of the many libraries and frameworks available in Python. The richness of the Python ecosystem allows developers to choose the tools that best fit their specific needs, whether they are building web applications, analyzing data, or working on cutting-edge AI projects.

2.4 PYTHON'S COMMUNITY TO LEARN

Python's success is based not solely on its features and libraries but also on its vibrant and welcoming community. The Python community is known for its inclusivity and supportiveness, making it an ideal environment for beginners and experts.

The Python Package Index, often called PyPI, is a central repository for Python packages and libraries. It hosts thousands of open-source packages that can be easily installed and used in Python projects using package managers like pip. This centralized repository simplifies the distribution and sharing of Python code.

Python enthusiasts gather at various conferences and events worldwide to learn, share knowledge, and network. PyCon, the largest annual Python conference, brings together developers, educators, and enthusiasts to discuss the latest trends and developments in the Python ecosystem.

Online communities and forums provide a platform for Python developers to seek help, share experiences, and collaborate on projects. Websites like Stack Overflow,

Reddit's/r/python, and Python-related subreddits are popular places to engage with the community.

Python Enhancement Proposals, or PEPs, are design documents that propose new features, improvements, or changes to the Python programming language. They are the mechanism by which the Python community discusses and decides on the language's future direction.

Python User Groups, or PUGs, are local communities of Python enthusiasts who meet regularly to discuss Python-related topics, share knowledge, and collaborate on projects. These groups exist in many cities worldwide, providing opportunities for in-person networking and learning.

Numerous books, online courses, and tutorials are available for learning Python. Python's approachable syntax makes it an excellent choice for teaching programming to beginners, and there are dedicated resources for educators and learners.

2.5 PYTHON'S IMPACT ON EDUCATION

Python's simplicity and readability have made it a popular choice for teaching programming to beginners, and it is widely used in educational institutions worldwide. Here are some reasons why Python is an excellent language for teaching:

Python's clean and straightforward syntax reduces the barrier to entry for beginners. It emphasizes using indentation for code structure, making it easy to understand and follow.

Python's versatility allows educators to teach various programming concepts, from fundamentals to advanced topics like data science, web development, and artificial intelligence.

A wealth of educational resources is available for Python, including textbooks, online courses, tutorials, and interactive coding platforms like Codecademy and Coursera.

Python's interactive shell (REPL) encourages experimentation and exploration. Students can immediately see the results of their code, which enhances the learning experience.

Python's use in industry and research makes it relevant to students' future careers. Learning Python equips them with valuable skills in demand in the job market.

2.6 PYTHON 2 VERSUS PYTHON 3

In Python 2, print was a statement, while in Python 3, it became a function. This change allowed for more flexibility and consistency in how printing is handled.

Python 3 embraced Unicode as the default string type, making it more robust for handling text data in different languages and character sets.

In Python 2, dividing two integers would perform integer division, truncating the result to an integer. Python 3 introduced the// operator for explicit integer division, while the/ operator performs floating-point division.

Python 3 introduced the range function as the default way to create iterable sequences of numbers. In Python 2, the range function generated lists, which could be memory-intensive for large ranges.

Python 3 introduced the print function, which offered more control over formatting and output. In Python 2, the print was a statement with limited formatting options.

Python 3 improved exception handling by introducing the keyword, allowing for better error handling and debugging.

It's essential to note that Python 2 is no longer maintained, and developers are strongly encouraged to migrate their code to Python 3 to benefit from the latest features, improvements, and security updates.

2.7 PYTHON'S ROLE IN DATA SCIENCE AND MACHINE LEARNING

Python's versatility and the availability of specialized libraries and frameworks have made it a dominant player in data science and machine learning. Data scientists and machine learning engineers commonly use Python for tasks such as data preprocessing, model development, and visualization. Here's how Python contributes to these fields:

Python libraries like pandas and NumPy simplify data preprocessing tasks, including data cleaning, transformation, and aggregation. Data scientists can efficiently handle large datasets and prepare them for analysis.

Python's machine learning libraries, such as scikit-learn, TensorFlow, and PyTorch, provide tools for building, training, and evaluating machine learning models. These libraries offer various algorithms for classification, regression, clustering, and more.

Deep learning, a subset of machine learning, has seen significant advancements with Python-based frameworks like TensorFlow and PyTorch. These frameworks enable developing deep neural networks for tasks like image recognition, natural language processing, and generative modeling.

Python's data visualization libraries, including Matplotlib, Seaborn, and Plotly, allow data scientists to create informative and visually appealing charts and graphs to communicate their findings effectively.

Jupyter notebooks provide an interactive environment for data exploration and analysis. They allow users to combine code, visualizations, and explanatory text in a single document, making it a valuable tool for data scientists and researchers.

Python's data science ecosystem is further enriched by libraries like SciPy (for scientific computing), StatsModels (for statistical modeling), and scikit-image (for image processing). These libraries extend Python's capabilities for specific data-related tasks.

Python's role in data science and machine learning continues to grow, driven by its user-friendly syntax, strong community support, and the availability of state-of-the-art tools and libraries.

2.8 CHALLENGES AND CONSIDERATIONS

While Python is a powerful and versatile language, it is not without its challenges and considerations:

Python's interpreted nature can result in slower execution speeds than languages like C++ or Java. However, this performance gap can often be mitigated through optimizations or native extensions.

The transition from Python 2 to Python 3 posed challenges for developers with legacy codebases. Ensuring that code is compatible with the latest Python version is essential for long-term maintainability.

Managing dependencies and packaging can be complex, especially when working on large projects with many external libraries. Tools like virtual environments and package managers help address these challenges.

While Python's syntax is beginner-friendly, mastering advanced concepts and libraries can be challenging. The learning curve may vary depending on a developer's background and the complexity of the tasks they wish to accomplish.

Python's extensive ecosystem can lead to fragmentation, with multiple libraries and frameworks offering similar functionality. Careful selection and documentation are essential to avoid confusion.

2.9 PYTHON BASICS

Let's begin with the basics of Python 3 with examples:

Variables and Data Types: In Python, you can declare variables without specifying their data types. Python automatically assigns the appropriate data type based on the value assigned to the variable. Here are some common data types:

```
# Integer
age = 25
# Floating-point number
height = 5.9
# String
name = "John"
# Boolean
is_student = True
```

Lists and Tuples: Lists and tuples store collections of items in Python. Lists are mutable (can be modified), while tuples are immutable (cannot be changed).

```
# List
fruits = ['apple', 'banana', 'cherry']
# Tuple
coordinates = (3, 4)
```

Control Flow: Python supports various control flow statements, including if, for, and while loops.

```
# If statement
if age >= 18:
    print("Adult.")
else:
    print("Minor.")
# For loop
for fruit in fruits:
    print(fruit)
# While loop
count = 0

while count < 5:
    print(count)
    count += 1
```

2.10 BUILT-IN PYTHON LIBRARIES

Python comes with a rich set of built-in libraries that provide essential functionalities for various programming tasks. These libraries are readily available, requiring no installation. Here are some of the most commonly used built-in Python libraries:

os: The os library provides a way to interact with the operating system. It allows you to perform operations like file and directory manipulation, environment variable management, and more.

```
import os
# List all files in the current directory
files = os.listdir('.')
for file in files:
    print(file)
```

sys: The sys library provides access to system-specific parameters and functions. It's commonly used for command-line arguments, exiting scripts, and interacting with the Python interpreter.

```
import sys
# Print command-line arguments
for arg in sys.argv:
    print(arg)
```

math: The math library offers a wide range of mathematical functions and constants, making it indispensable for mathematical calculations.

```
import math
x = 25
sqrt_x = math.sqrt(x)
print(f"The square root of {x} is {sqrt_x}")
```

The square root of 25 is 5.0

random: The random library provides functions for generating random numbers and performing randomization tasks. Example: Rolling a Six-Sided Die

```python
import random
# Generate a random number between 1 and 6 (inclusive)
roll = random.randint(1, 6)
print(f"You rolled a {roll}")
```

You rolled a 5

datetime: The datetime library allows for working with dates and times, making it useful for tasks involving time-based calculations and formatting.

Example: Displaying the Current Date and Time

```python
import datetime
now = datetime.datetime.now()
print(f"Current date and time: {now}")
```

Current date and time: 2023-10-09 11:03:19.873707

2.11 DATA MANIPULATION LIBRARIES

Data manipulation is fundamental to many Python applications, particularly in data science and analysis. Several libraries excel in this domain, enabling efficient data handling, processing, and visualization.

2.11.1 NumPy

NumPy is a fundamental library in Python for numerical and scientific computing. It is an open-source project that supports large, multi-dimensional arrays and matrices, along with a collection of mathematical functions to operate on these arrays efficiently. NumPy is built on top of the Python programming language and is an essential tool in various fields such as data science, machine learning, physics, engineering, and more.

NumPy offers several advantages that make it a preferred choice for numerical computation:

- NumPy's core functionality is implemented in C and Fortran, making it highly efficient for numerical operations. This efficiency is crucial for handling large datasets and performing complex mathematical calculations.

- NumPy introduces the ndarray (N-dimensional array) data structure, which allows you to work with multi-dimensional data effortlessly. This is especially useful for tasks like image processing, signal processing, and simulations.

- NumPy provides a wide range of mathematical functions, including basic operations, linear algebra, Fourier transforms, and more. These functions are optimized for performance and can be applied to entire arrays without the need for explicit loops.

- NumPy seamlessly integrates with other scientific libraries, such as SciPy (for scientific computing), Matplotlib (for data visualization), and scikit-learn (for machine learning). This ecosystem makes Python a powerful platform for scientific and data analysis.

Installing NumPy: Before we dive into NumPy, let's make sure you have it installed. You can install NumPy using pip, the Python package manager: **pip install numpy**

Once installed, you can import NumPy into your Python code: **import numpy as np**

Now that we have NumPy installed and imported, let's move on to the basics of NumPy arrays.

At the core of NumPy is the ndarray (N-dimensional array) data structure. This is the primary container for numerical data in NumPy and provides efficient storage and operations on large datasets.

NumPy arrays have the following important attributes:

- Shape: The dimensions of the array, specified as a tuple of integers.

- dtype: The data type of the elements in the array, such as integers, floating-point numbers, etc.

- Strides: Information about how the elements are stored in memory for efficient access.

Let's start by creating a simple NumPy array:

```python
import numpy as np
# Create a 1D array
arr = np.array([1-5])
print(arr)
```

[1 2 3 4 5]

np.zeros() and np.ones(): You can create arrays filled with zeros or ones using np.zeros() and np.ones(), respectively.

```python
 Create an array of zeros
zeros_arr = np.zeros((3, 4))
print(zeros_arr)
# Create an array of ones
ones_arr = np.ones((2, 3))
print(ones_arr)
```

```
[[0., 0., 0., 0.],
  [0., 0., 0., 0.],
  [0., 0., 0., 0.]]

 [[1., 1., 1.],
  [1., 1., 1.]]
```

np.arange(): It generates an array of evenly spaced values within a given range.

```
# Create an array of values from 0 to 9
range_arr = np.arange(10)
print(range_arr)

# Create an array of values from 2 to 8
range_arr2 = np.arange(2, 9)
print(range_arr2)

[0, 1, 2, 3, 4, 5, 6, 7, 8, 9]
[2-8]
```

np.linspace(): It generates an array of evenly spaced values over a specified range.

```
linspace _ arr = np.linspace(0, 1, 5)
print(linspace_arr)

 [0. , 0.25, 0.5 , 0.75, 1. ]
```

np.random: NumPy also provides functions for generating random arrays. Here are a few examples:

```
# Create a random 2x2 array with values between 0 and 1
random_arr = np.random.rand(2, 2)
print(random_arr)

[[0.81573922 0.35474141]
 [0.84329603 0.27445619]]

# Create a random 2x2 array with values from a standard normal
distribution
normal_arr = np.random.randn(2, 2)
print(normal_arr)

[[ 0.5221833   0.22731988]
 [-0.26163641 -1.00853621]]
```

Concatenating Arrays: You can concatenate arrays vertically or horizontally using np.concatenate() and related functions.

```
# Create two arrays
arr1 = np.array([1-3])
arr2 = np.array([4-6])
```

```
# Concatenate vertically
concatenated_vert = np.concatenate((arr1, arr2))
print("Concatenated Vertically:", concatenated_vert)

# Concatenate horizontally
concatenated_horiz = np.vstack((arr1, arr2))
print("Concatenated Horizontally:")
print(concatenated_horiz)

Concatenated Vertically: [1 2 3 4 5 6]
Concatenated Horizontally:
[[1 2 3]
 [4 5 6]]
```

Mathematical Functions: You can perform various mathematical operations elementwise on arrays using NumPy's vectorized functions.

```
# Create an array
arr = np.array([1-5])

# Square root of each element
sqrt_arr = np.sqrt(arr)
print("Square Root:", sqrt_arr)

# Exponential function
exp_arr = np.exp(arr)
print("Exponential:", exp_arr)

# Element-wise logarithm
log_arr = np.log(arr)
print("Logarithm:", log_arr)

Square Root: [1.         1.41421356 1.73205081 2.         2.23606798]
Exponential: [  2.71828183   7.3890561   20.08553692  54.59815003
148.4131591 ]
Logarithm: [0.         0.69314718 1.09861229 1.38629436 1.60943791]
```

NumPy and Linear Algebra: NumPy provides comprehensive support for linear algebra operations, making it a valuable tool for scientific and engineering applications. Matrix multiplication can be performed using the dot() function or the @ operator.

```
# Create two matrices
A = np.array([[1, 2], [3, 4]])
B = np.array([[5, 6], [7, 8]])

# Matrix multiplication
result = A.dot(B)
print("Matrix Multiplication:\n", result)

[[19 22]
 [43 50]]
```

Eigenvalues and Eigenvectors: You can compute the eigenvalues and eigenvectors of a matrix using NumPy.

```
# Create an Array
A = np.array([[2, -1], [-1, 3]])
# Compute eigenvalues and eigenvectors
eigenvalues, eigenvectors = np.linalg.eig(A)
print("Eigenvalues:", eigenvalues)
print("Eigenvectors:\n", eigenvectors)
```

```
Eigenvalues: [1.38196601 3.61803399]
Eigenvectors:
 [[-0.85065081  0.52573111]
 [-0.52573111 -0.85065081]]
```

Solving Linear Equations: NumPy can solve systems of linear equations using the numpy.linalg.solve() function.

```
# Define the coefficients matrix A and the right-hand side vector b
A = np.array([[2, 3], [1, -2]])
b = np.array([1, 8])
# Solve the linear system Ax = b
x = np.linalg.solve(A, b)
print("Solution:", x)
```

```
Solution: [2.71428571 0.85714286]
```

Handling Missing Data: NumPy provides tools for handling missing data, often represented as np.nan (Not-a-Number).

```
# Create an array with missing values
arr = np.array([1, 2, np.nan, 4, 5])
# Check for missing values
has_nan = np.isnan(arr)
print("Missing Values:", has_nan)
# Replace missing values with a specific value
arr[has_nan] = 0
print("Array with Missing Values Replaced:\n", arr)
```

```
Missing Values: [False False  True False False]
Array with Missing Values Replaced:
[1. 2. 0. 4. 5.]
```

Filtering and Sorting Data: You can filter data in NumPy arrays and sort the elements based on conditions.

```
# Create an array
arr = np.array([1-6, 9])
# Filter values greater than 3
filtered_arr = arr[arr > 3]
```

```
print("Filtered Array:", filtered_arr)
# Sort the array
sorted_arr = np.sort(arr)
print("Sorted Array:", sorted_arr)
```

```
Filtered Array: [4 5 9 6 5]
Sorted Array: [1 1 2 3 3 4 5 5 6 9]
```

2.11.2 Statistical Analysis

NumPy provides functions for basic statistical analysis, such as mean, median, variance, and standard deviation.

```
# Create an array
arr = np.array([1-5])
# Calculate mean
mean_val = np.mean(arr)
print("Mean:", mean_val)
# Calculate median
median_val = np.median(arr)
print("Median:", median_val)
# Calculate variance
variance_val = np.var(arr)
print("Variance:", variance_val)
# Calculate standard deviation
std_deviation_val = np.std(arr)
print("Standard Deviation:", std_deviation_val)
```

```
Mean: 3.0
Median: 3.0
Variance: 2.0
Standard Deviation: 1.4142135623730951
```

Many machines learning libraries, including scikit-learn and TensorFlow, rely on NumPy for data storage and manipulation. NumPy arrays are the preferred data structure for training and evaluating machine learning models. Below is an example of how NumPy is used in this regard. Later chapter about machine learning will discuss more about machine learning codes in Python. In the following example, LinearRegression machine learning model is applied for training some data created by numpy array and later a random test data is used for prediction. Here X is training data and y training categories. Test_X is testing data applied on the trained model for prediction.

```
from sklearn.linear_model import LinearRegression
# Create synthetic data
X = np.array([[1, 2], [2, 3], [3, 4]])
y = np.array([3, 5, 7])
# Create a linear regression model
```

```
model = LinearRegression()
# Train the model
model.fit(X, y)
# Make predictions
predictions = model.predict(X)
#Predicting trained data
print("Predicting trained data ", predictions)
#Test data
Test_X = np.array([[1, 3],])
#Predicting test data
print("Predicting test data ", model.predict(Test_X))

Predicting trained data   [3. 5. 7.]
Predicting test data   [4.]
```

2.12 PANDAS

Pandas is an open-source Python library designed for data manipulation and analysis. Pandas provides data structures and functions that simplify working with structured data, making it an essential tool for data cleaning, transformation, and exploration. Pandas offers several key benefits for data analysis:

- Pandas introduces two primary data structures, the Series and DataFrame, which are powerful tools for handling structured data.

- It provides functions to handle missing data, filter and clean datasets, and perform data transformation tasks efficiently.

- Pandas enables data exploration through various methods for summarizing, aggregating, and visualizing data.

- It supports data loading and saving from various file formats, including CSV, Excel, and more.

- Pandas can handle a wide range of data types, making it suitable for both small and large datasets.

- Pandas can be seamlessly integrated with other Python libraries such as NumPy, Matplotlib, and scikit-learn.

To install Pandas, you can use pip, the Python package manager. Open your command prompt or terminal and run the following command:

pip install pandas

Once installed, you can import Pandas into your Python script or Jupyter Notebook using:

import pandas as pd

2.12.1 Pandas Data Structures

Pandas provides three primary data structures for working with data: Series, DataFrame, and Index.

A Series is a one-dimensional array-like object that can hold various data types, including integers, floats, strings, and more. It is similar to a column in a spreadsheet or a single variable in statistics. You can create a Series from a list or array, like this:

```
import pandas as pd
data = [1-5]
series = pd.Series(data)
```

A DataFrame is a two-dimensional table-like data structure with rows and columns. It is similar to a spreadsheet or a SQL table and is the most commonly used Pandas data structure. You can create a DataFrame from various data sources, such as a dictionary, a CSV file, or a SQL query result. Here's an example of creating a DataFrame from a dictionary:

```
data = {
    'Name': ['Alice', 'Bob', 'Charlie'],
    'Age': [25, 30, 35]
}
df = pd.DataFrame(data)
```

An Index is an immutable array that labels the rows or columns in a DataFrame. It allows for efficient data retrieval and alignment. By default, DataFrames have row labels (index) and column labels. You can also set custom labels for better data management.

```
data = {'A': [1-3], 'B': [4-6]}
df = pd.DataFrame(data, index=['X', 'Y', 'Z'])
```

In this example, 'X', 'Y', and 'Z' are custom row labels.

2.12.2 Basic Operations

Now that we have an understanding of Pandas data structures, let's explore some basic operations you can perform with them. Before diving into data analysis, it's essential to understand your dataset. Pandas provides several methods for inspecting your data:

You can use the head() and tail() methods to display the first or last few rows of a DataFrame:

```
df.head()    # Displays the first 5 rows by default
df.tail(3)   # Displays the last 3 rows
```

Use the info() method to get a summary of the DataFrame, including the data types, non-null values, and memory usage:

```
df.info()
```

Pandas offers the describe() method to generate summary statistics for numeric columns:

```
df.describe()
```

You can access specific data within a DataFrame or Series using various methods:

```
df['Name']   # Selects the 'Name' column
df.Age  # Equivalent to df['Age']
```

To select multiple columns, use double square brackets:

```
df[['Name', 'Age']]   # Selects both 'Name' and 'Age' columns
```

You can select rows by using the loc[] or iloc[] indexer:

```
df.loc['X']   # Selects the row with index 'X'
df.iloc[1]   # Selects the second row (index 1)
```

You can filter data based on conditions using Boolean indexing:

```
df[df['Age'] > 30]   # Selects rows where 'Age' is greater than 30
```

You can create a new column and assign values to it:

```
df['Salary'] = [50000, 60000, 70000]
```

To modify data in a DataFrame, use assignment:

```
df.loc['X', 'Age'] = 26  # Change the age of 'X' to 26
```

You can drop rows or columns using the drop() method:

```
df.drop('X', inplace=True)   # Removes the row with index 'X'
df.drop('Salary', axis=1, inplace=True)   # Removes the 'Salary'
column
```

Pandas provides methods to handle missing data, represented as NaN (Not a Number): Use the isna() or isnull() method to check for missing values:

```
df.isna()   # Returns a DataFrame of True/False indicating missing
values
df.isna().sum()   # Counts missing values in each column
```

You can remove rows with missing data using dropna():

```
df.dropna()   # Removes rows with any missing values
```

Use fillna() to fill missing values with a specified value or method:

```
df.fillna(0)   # Fills missing values with 0
df.fillna(df.mean())   # Fills missing values with the mean of the
column
```

You can read data from CSV, Excel, SQL databases, and more using Pandas' read_ functions. Here's an example line of code of reading data from a CSV file, writing data to a CSV file, and writing data to an Excel file.

```
df = pd.read_csv('data.csv')
df.to_csv('output.csv', index=False)  # Save to CSV without the index
df.to_excel('output.xlsx', sheet_name='Sheet1', index=False)  #
Save to Excel
```

You can filter rows based on conditions using Boolean indexing. For example, the following example filter the rows with salary is higher than 50,000

```
high_income = df[df['Salary'] > 50000]  # Filter rows where salary
is > 50000
```

Sort your data using the sort_values() method:

```
df.sort_values(by='Age', ascending=False)  # Sort by 'Age' in
descending order
```

You can group data and perform aggregations using the groupby() method:

```
grouped = df.groupby('Department')
grouped['Salary'].mean()  # Calculate the mean salary per department
```

Combine DataFrames using methods like concat(), merge(), or join():

```
df1 = pd.DataFrame({'A': [1, 2], 'B': [3, 4]})
df2 = pd.DataFrame({'A': [5, 6], 'B': [7, 8]})
result = pd.concat([df1, df2])  # Concatenate DataFrames
```

2.13 DATA VISUALIZATION

Data visualization is a powerful way to communicate insights and patterns from your data. In Python, you have access to several libraries that make data visualization a breeze. Some of the most popular libraries include Matplotlib, Seaborn, and Plotly. Let's explore each of them with some example code:

2.13.1 Matplotlib

Matplotlib is a fundamental data visualization library in Python. It provides a wide range of customizable plots and charts. Matplotlib offers extensive customization options to make your plots more informative and visually appealing. Here are some common customizations as shown in following codes. Figures 2.1 and 2.2 show different plots of data using the Matplotlib library.

```
import matplotlib.pyplot as plt
x = [1–5]
y = [10, 12, 5, 8, 15]
```

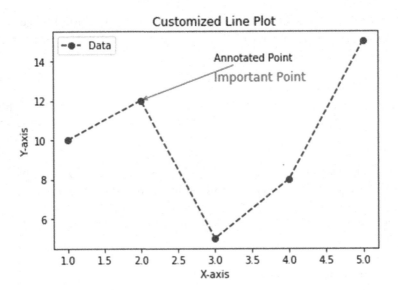

FIGURE 2.1   Matplotlib example to draw customized line plot.

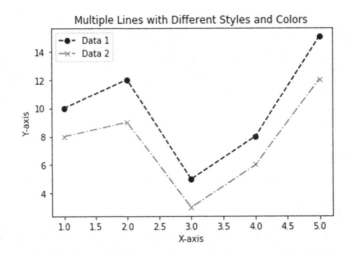

FIGURE 2.2   Matplotlib example to draw multiple lines with multiple styles.

```
plt.plot(x, y, marker='o', linestyle='--', color='b', label='Data')
plt.xlabel('X-axis')
plt.ylabel('Y-axis')
plt.title('Customized Line Plot')

# Adding text and an arrow annotation
plt.text(3, 13, 'Important Point', fontsize=12, color='red')
plt.annotate('Annotated Point', xy=(2, 12), xytext=(3, 14),
            arrowprops=dict(arrowstyle='->', color='green'))

plt.legend()
plt.show()
```

```
import matplotlib.pyplot as plt

x = [1-5]
y1 = [10, 12, 5, 8, 15]
y2 = [8, 9, 3, 6, 12]

plt.plot(x, y1, marker='o', linestyle='--', color='b', label='Data 1')
plt.plot(x, y2, marker='x', linestyle='-.', color='r', label='Data 2')
plt.xlabel('X-axis')
plt.ylabel('Y-axis')
plt.title('Multiple Lines with Different Styles and Colors')
plt.legend()
plt.show()

ax.scatter(x, y, z, c='b', marker='o')
ax.set_xlabel('X-axis')
ax.set_ylabel('Y-axis')
ax.set_zlabel('Z-axis')
ax.set_title('3D Scatter Plot')
```

2.13.2 Seaborn

Seaborn is built on top of Matplotlib and offers a higher-level interface for creating stylish statistical visualizations. We covered customizing Matplotlib plots and advanced techniques for creating more complex visualizations. In this part, we'll dive into Seaborn, a powerful data visualization library built on top of Matplotlib. Seaborn provides a higher-level interface for creating stylish statistical visualizations. Figure 2.3 shows a pair plot for exploring relationships between variables of iris dataset available in the Seaborn library of Python. The iris dataset, a classic benchmark in machine learning, is often visualized using Seaborn in Python. Seaborn simplifies data exploration by providing aesthetically pleasing statistical graphics. With its concise syntax, Seaborn allows users to effortlessly create informative plots, facilitating comprehensive analysis and visualization of the iris dataset's botanical attributes and species classification. Let's further explore different features of *seaborn* using following code journey.

```
import seaborn as sns
import matplotlib.pyplot as plt
# Load a sample dataset
iris = sns.load_dataset('iris')

# Create a pair plot for exploring relationships between variables
sns.pairplot(iris, hue='species')
plt.show()
```

We can show a heatmap (i.e., Figure 2.4) as follows:

```
import seaborn as sns
import matplotlib.pyplot as plt
# Create a heatmap to visualize the correlation matrix
correlation_matrix = iris.corr()
```

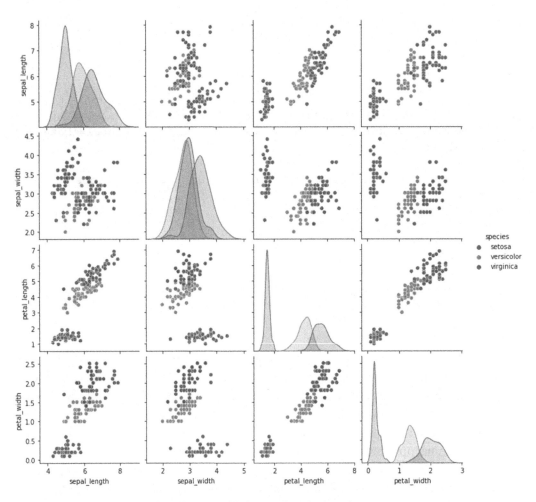

FIGURE 2.3   Seaborn example to draw multiple lines with multiple styles.

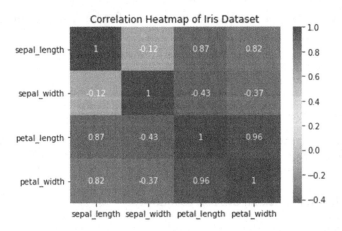

FIGURE 2.4   Seaborn example to show correlation between attributes.

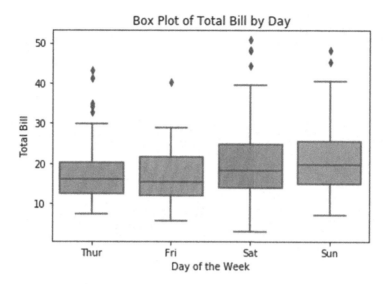

FIGURE 2.5   Seaborn example to show box plots of attributes.

```
sns.heatmap(correlation_matrix, annot=True, cmap="coolwarm")
plt.title('Correlation Heatmap of Iris Dataset')
plt.show()
```

We can show a box plot (i.e., Figure 2.5) as follows:

```
import seaborn as sns
import matplotlib.pyplot as plt
# Load a sample dataset
tips = sns.load_dataset('tips')

# Create a box plot to visualize the distribution of total bills
sns.boxplot(x='day', y='total_bill', data=tips, palette='Set2')
plt.xlabel('Day of the Week')
plt.ylabel('Total Bill')
plt.title('Box Plot of Total Bill by Day')
plt.show()
```

We can show a scatter plot (i.e., Figure 2.6) as follows:

```
import seaborn as sns
import matplotlib.pyplot as plt
# Load a sample dataset
tips = sns.load_dataset('tips')
sns.scatterplot(data=tips, x="total_bill", y="tip")
```

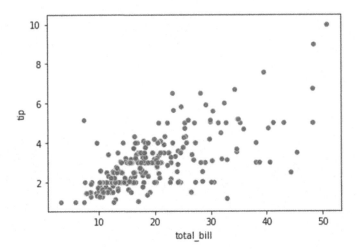

Figure 2.6   Seaborn example to show scatterplot of attributes.

2.14 CONCLUSION

This chapter provides basic ideas about Python and its different important libraries to explore data and visualize it. Simple examples have been included to show the results of small segments of codes so that they can be used for any dataset when needed for different datasets. Python continues to be a prominent programming language, leaving a lasting impact on software development and data science. Python's emphasis on simplicity, readability, and flexibility has garnered among programmers, regardless of their experience level. The language's extensive library ecosystem encompasses tools like NumPy, Pandas, and Matplotlib for data analysis. Python's open-source nature and the robust developer community have fostered a collaborative atmosphere, creating numerous free packages, frameworks, and tools. This thriving ecosystem has positioned Python as a leader in emerging fields such as artificial intelligence, data science, and automation. Python's enduring relevance underscores its adaptability, accessibility, and wide-ranging applicability across numerous industries, reaffirming its status as a cornerstone of modern software development. As technology advances, Python remains poised to evolve and innovate, meeting the evolving demands of the digital era.

REFERENCES

[1] R. Mastrodomenico, *The Python Book*, John Wiley & Sons Ltd, 2022, doi: 10.1002/9781119573364

[2] W. McKinney, *Python for Data Analysis*, O'Reilly Media, 2021.

[3] P. Deitel and H. Deitel, *Intro to Python for Computer Science and Data Science: Learning to Program with AI, Big Data and the Cloud*, Prentice-Hall, 2020.

[4] A. Sweigart, *Automate the Boring Stuff with Python: Practical Programming for Total Beginners*, No Starch Press, 2020.

[5] E. Matthes, *Python Crash Course*, No Starch Press, 2021.

[6] E. B. Matloff, *Python for Data Science*, CRC Press, 2020.

[7] C. Severance, *Python for Everybody: Exploring Data Using Python 3*, Charles Severance, 2021.

[8] M. Lutz, *Learning Python*, O'Reilly Media, 2013.

[9] M. F. Lane, *Python Machine Learning*, Packt Publishing, 2020.

[10] D. Golding, *Beginning Programming with Python For Dummies*, John Wiley & Sons, 2020.

## CHAPTER 3

Feature Analysis Using Python

3.1 FEATURE EXTRACTION

Features can be defined as functions of essential attributes that define some quantitative properties of an event or object. These functions are often helpful for classification or pattern recognition. It is necessary to know that a good representation of data in a particular domain for specific tasks depends on the number of measurements available. Current applications employ various features, which can be classified into low-level and high-level features. The classification of low-level and high-level features remains unclear as there is as yet no specific or clear guideline. In general, obtaining high-level features is more challenging than deriving low-level features. Low-level features are fundamental characteristics directly derived from the data without much description. Conversely, the high-level feature involves finding shapes and objects in computer images at a high-level description. Several low-level features form the basis of high-level features. Low-level features include general features as well as local features. General features typically consist of raw data, but are based on application-independent features. Local features are computed based on a subdivision of the data. Features computed by high-level feature algorithms are calculated from the entire data of an event or even a regular portion of the data. Automated feature extraction techniques can replace the human expertise necessary for converting raw data into valuable features manually by replacing the need for human expertise. In the feature extraction process, raw data is transformed into a form that represents the informational characteristics of a system. This will enable the representation of information efficiently, which can benefit classification and analysis. Research involving pattern recognition or classification usually consists of applying a specific form of dimensionality reduction when evaluating feature extraction. A decrease in the representation of features is achieved by removing redundant information from input data, which has high dimensions and can be challenging to process. This reduction of representation is referred to as feature vectors, which are reduced representation sets of features. Based on the fact that the extracted features were selected to enable them to extract the relevant information to accomplish the desired task using reduced dimensional information, it is hoped that the features will extract accurate information.

DOI: 10.1201/9781003425908-3

3.2 PRINCIPAL COMPONENT ANALYSIS (PCA)

The Principal Component Analysis (PCA) method widely approximates the original data within a lower-dimensional feature space [1–20]. An approximation is performed by computing the top eigenvectors of the covariance data matrix Q and then combining them linearly. As indicated below, the covariance matrix for the sample training image vectors and the covariance matrix PCs can each be calculated as follows:

$$Q = \frac{1}{T} \sum_{i=1}^{T} \left(\tilde{X}_i \tilde{X}_i^T \right)$$
$$E^T Q E = \Lambda$$

where E represents the matrix of orthonormal eigenvectors and the diagonal matrix of the eigenvalues. This reflects the original coordinate system onto the eigenvectors where the eigenvector corresponding to the largest eigenvalue indicates the axis of most considerable variance and the next largest one is the orthogonal axis of the largest one, indicating the second most significant variance. A subspace can be defined using several eigenvectors that correspond to the largest eigenvalues since the variance is negligible for eigenvalues that are close to zero. This allows the full-dimensional data to be represented easily in a reduced dimension. Figure 3.1 illustrates two principal components that account for the majority of the variance in data.

```
Import matplotlib. pyplot as plt
import mpl_toolkits.mplot3d
import numpy as np

from sklearn import datasets, decomposition

np.random.seed(5)

iris = datasets.load _ iris()
X = iris.data
y = iris.target
```

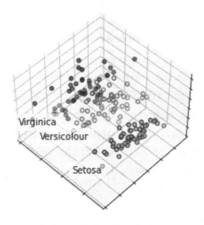

FIGURE 3.1   Principal Component Analysis applied to the iris dataset.

```
fig = plt.figure(1, figsize=(4, 3))
plt.clf()

ax = fig.add _ subplot(111, projection="3d", elev=48, azim=134)
ax.set_position([0, 0, 0.95, 1])

plt.cla()
pca = decomposition.PCA(n_components=3)
pca.fit(X)
X = pca.transform(X)

for name, label in [("Setosa", 0), ("Versicolour", 1), ("Virginica", 2)]:
    ax.text3D(
        X[y == label, 0].mean(),
        X[y == label, 1].mean() + 1.5,
        X[y == label, 2].mean(),
        name,
        horizontalalignment="center",
        bbox=dict(alpha=0.5, edgecolor="w", facecolor="w"),
    )
# Reorder the labels to have colors matching the cluster results
y = np.choose(y, [1, 2, 0]).astype(float)
ax.scatter(X[:, 0], X[:, 1], X[:, 2], c=y, cmap=plt.cm.nipy_
spectral, edgecolor="k")

ax.xaxis.set _ ticklabels([])
ax.yaxis.set_ticklabels([])
ax.zaxis.set_ticklabels([])

plt.show()
```

3.3 KERNEL PRINCIPAL COMPONENT ANALYSIS (KPCA)

The typical PCA method follows a linear structure to locate the directions resulting in the maximum variation, making it difficult to characterize nonlinear data. Kernel-based Principal Component Analysis (i.e., KPCA) can be employed to overcome such limitations [21–27]. In KPCA, input features are transformed into a higher-dimensional feature space by using a kernel (e.g., Gaussian). Using this high-dimensional feature space, typical PCA is performed. Given data X, the covariance C of the M can be represented as

$$C = \frac{1}{N} \sum_{i=1}^{N} \left(\Theta(X_i) . \Theta(X_i)^T \right),$$

$$\Theta(X_i) = \Phi(X_i) - \bar{\Phi},$$

$$\bar{\Phi} = \frac{1}{N} \sum_{i=1}^{N} \Phi(X_i)$$

where N represents the total number of data and Φ is a kernel. Then, eigenvalue decomposition is done on the covariance matrix to find the principal components as

$$\lambda E = CE,$$
$$C = E^T \lambda E$$

where E represents eigenvectors (i.e., principal components) and λ eigenvalues. The feature vectors using KPCA on the data X can be represented as

$$P_{\text{KPCA}} = XE_m$$

where m is the top m principal component. A similar projection can also be applied to a typical PCA. Figure 3.2 shows samples of two classes from a dataset available under the *sklearn* library. Figure 3.3 shows the samples after applying PCA. Figure 3.4 shows the KPCA projection on the same samples which indicates that it is possible to separate them after applying KPCA.

```
import matplotlib.pyplot as plt
from sklearn.datasets import make_moons
X, y = make_moons(100, random_state=123)
plt.scatter(X[y==0, 0], X[y==0, 1],color='red', marker='^',
alpha=0.5)
plt.scatter(X[y==1, 0], X[y==1, 1],color='blue', marker='o',
alpha=0.5)
plt.tight_layout()
plt.show()
```

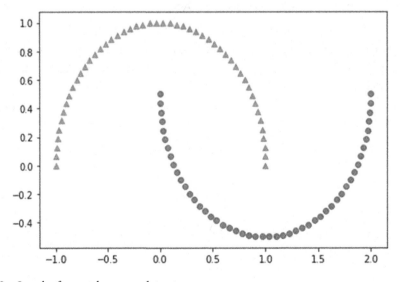

FIGURE 3.2   Samples from make moons dataset.

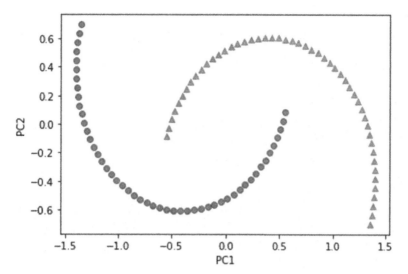

FIGURE 3.3   PCA projections on samples from make moons dataset.

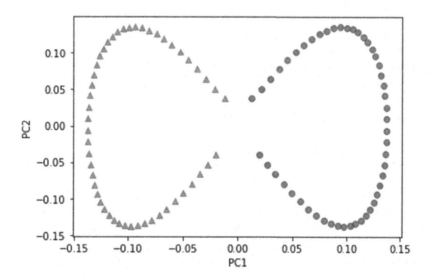

FIGURE 3.4   KPCA projections on samples from make moons dataset.

```
from sklearn.decomposition import PCA
scikit_pca = PCA(n_components=2)
X_spca = scikit_pca.fit_transform(X)
plt.scatter(X_kpca[y==0, 0], X_kpca[y==0, 1],color='red',
marker='^', alpha=0.5)
plt.scatter(X_kpca[y==1, 0], X_kpca[y==1, 1],color='blue',
marker='o', alpha=0.5)
plt.xlabel('PC1')
```

```python
plt.ylabel('PC2')
plt.show()

From scipy.spatial.distance import pdist, squareform
from scipy import exp
from scipy.linalg import eigh
import numpy as np
def rbf_kernel_pca(X, gamma, n_components):
    """
    RBF kernel PCA implementation.
    Parameters
    ------------
    X: {NumPy ndarray}, shape = [n_examples, n_features]
    gamma: float
        Tuning parameter of the RBF kernel
    n_components: int
        Number of principal components to return
    Returns
    ------------
    X_pc: {NumPy ndarray}, shape = [n_examples, k_features]
        Projected dataset
    """
    # Calculate pairwise squared Euclidean distances
    # in the MxN dimensional dataset.
    Sq_dists = pdist(X, 'sqeuclidean')
    # Convert pairwise distances into a square matrix.
    Mat_sq_dists = squareform(sq_dists)
    # Compute the symmetric kernel matrix.
    K = exp(-gamma * mat_sq_dists)
    # Center the kernel matrix.
    N = K.shape[0]
    one_n = np.ones((N,N)) / N
    K = K - one_n.dot(K) - K.dot(one_n) + one_n.dot(K).dot(one_n)
    # Obtaining eigenpairs from the centered kernel matrix
    # scipy.linalg.eigh returns them in ascending order
    eigvals, eigvecs = eigh(K)
    eigvals, eigvecs = eigvals[::-1], eigvecs[:, ::-1]
    # Collect the top k eigenvectors (projected examples)
    X_pc = np.column_stack([eigvecs[:, i]
                            for I in range(n_components)])
    return X_pca

X_kpca = rbf_kernel_pca(X, gamma=15, n_components=2)
plt.scatter(X_kpca[y==0, 0], X_kpca[y==0, 1],color='red',
marker='^', alpha=0.5)
plt.scatter(X_kpca[y==1, 0], X_kpca[y==1, 1],color='blue',
marker='o', alpha=0.5)
plt.xlabel('PC1')
plt.ylabel('PC2')
plt.show()
```

3.4 FEATURE EXTRACTION USING ICA

This addresses the difficulty of finding statistically independent basis sources between variables [28–48]. The basic principle of Independent Component Analysis (ICA) is to use a basis function to represent observations with independent components. If S is a collection of basis images and X is a collection of input images, then the relation between X and S is modeled as

$$X = MS$$

where M represents an unknown linear mixing matrix of full rank.

An ICA algorithm learns the weight matrix W, which is the inverse of the mixing matrix M. W is used to recover a set of independent basis images. The ICA basis vectors focus on extracting local feature information rather than global as in PCA. ICA basis vectors represent the local feature data. Before applying ICA, PCA can be used to reduce the dimension of the data, which is typically known as enhanced ICA. Thus, ICA is performed on data vectors as follows.

$$S = WE^T$$

$$E^T = W^{-1}S$$

$$X_r = VW^{-1}S$$

where V is projection of the data X on E_m and X_r the reconstructed original data. The feature vectors using ICA on the data X can be represented as

$$P_{ICA} = XE_mW^{-1}$$

where m is the top m principal components. Figure 3.5 shows the essence of ICA to represent independent non-orthogonal sources rather than PCA that typical represents orthogonal components.

An example of estimating sources from noisy data. Independent Component A estimates sources given noisy measurements. Imagine three instruments playing simultaneously and three microphones recording the mixed signals. ICA is used to recover the sources i.e. what is played by each instrument. Importantly, PCA fails at recovering since the related signals reflect non-Gaussian processes.

```
import numpy as np
from scipy import signal

np.random.seed(0)
n_samples = 2000
time = np.linspace(0, 8, n_samples)
```

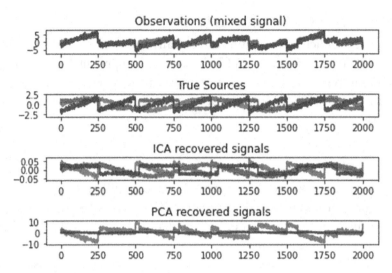

FIGURE 3.5 PCA versus ICA.

```python
s1 = np.sin(2 * time)  # Signal 1 : sinusoidal signal
s2 = np.sign(np.sin(3 * time))  # Signal 2 : square signal
s3 = signal.sawtooth(2 * np.pi * time)  # Signal 3: saw tooth
signal

S = np.c _ [s1, s2, s3]
S += 0.2 * np.random.normal(size=S.shape)  # Add noise

S /= S.std(axis=0)  # Standardize data
# Mix data
A = np.array([[1, 1, 1], [0.5, 2, 1.0], [1.5, 1.0, 2.0]])  #
Mixing matrix
X = np.dot(S, A.T)  # Generate observations


from sklearn.decomposition import PCA, FastICA
# Compute ICA
ica = FastICA(n_components=3, whiten="arbitrary-variance")
S_ = ica.fit_transform(X)  # Reconstruct signals
A_ = ica.mixing_  # Get estimated mixing matrix

# We can `prove` that the ICA model applies by reverting the unmixing.
assert np.allclose(X, np.dot(S_, A_.T) + ica.mean_)

# For comparison, compute PCA
pca = PCA(n_components=3)
H = pca.fit_transform(X)  # Reconstruct signals based on
orthogonal components

import matplotlib.pyplot as plt

plt.figure()
```

```
models = [X, S, S _ , H]
names = [
    "Observations (mixed signal)",
    "True Sources",
    "ICA recovered signals",
    "PCA recovered signals",
]
colors = ["red", "green", "blue"]

for ii, (model, name) in enumerate(zip(models, names), 1):
    plt.subplot(4, 1, ii)
    plt.title(name)
    for sig, color in zip(model.T, colors):
        plt.plot(sig, color=color)

plt.tight _ layout()
plt.show()
```

3.5 LINEAR DISCRIMINANT ANALYSIS (LDA)

Linear Discriminant Analysis (LDA) produces an optimal linear discriminant function which maps the input into the classification space based on which the class identification of the samples can be decided [49–66]. The within-scatter matrix, S_W and the between-scatter matrix, S_B are computed by the following equations:

$$S_B = \sum_{i=1}^{c} G_i \left(\overline{m}_i - \overline{\overline{m}} \right)\left(\overline{m}_i - \overline{\overline{m}} \right)^T$$

$$S_W = \sum_{i=1}^{c} \sum_{m_k \in C_i} \left(m_k - \overline{m}_i \right)\left(m_k - \overline{m}_i \right)^T$$

where G_i is the number of vectors in i^{th} class C_i. c is the number of classes and, in our case, it represents the number of classes. $\overline{\overline{m}}$ represents the mean of all vectors, $\overline{m}_i$ the mean of the class C_i and m_k the vector of a specific class. The optimal discrimination feature matrix D_{LDA} is chosen from the maximization of ratio of the determinant of the between and within-class scatter matrix as

$$D_{\text{LDA}} = \arg\max_{D} \frac{\left| D^T S_B D \right|}{\left| D^T S_W D \right|}$$

where D_{LDA} is the set of discriminant vectors of S_W and S_B corresponding to the $(c - 1)$ largest generalized eigenvalues λ and can be obtained via solving

$$S_B d_i = \lambda_i S_W d_i.$$

Using LDA, the extracted data representations from different classes can then be extended by LDA to produce the best discrimination among classes. So, the LDA algorithm seeks out vectors in the underlying space that create the best discrimination among different **classes**. LDA can be used to generate feature vectors as follows:

$$P_{\text{LDA}} = XD_{\text{LDA}}^T.$$

Figure 3.6 shows PCA versus LDA projection on some data from famous iris dataset [67] where LDA represents better class separation for the example two classes. The figures related to features have been generated using the scikit-learn machine learning library [67]. Figure 2.6 shows sample code segments to build feature spaces and projection of data on to them for different feature extraction techniques using scikit-learn.

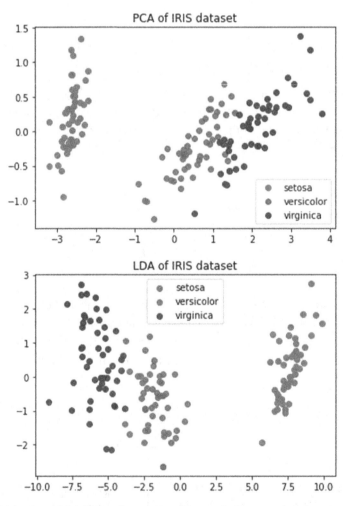

FIGURE 3.6   PCA (top) and LDA (bottom) projections on samples from iris dataset.

```
import matplotlib.pyplot as plt

from sklearn import datasets
from sklearn.decomposition import PCA
from sklearn.discriminant_analysis import
LinearDiscriminantAnalysis

iris = datasets.load _ iris()

X = iris.data
y = iris.target
target_names = iris.target_names

pca = PCA(n _ components=2)
X_r = pca.fit(X).transform(X)

lda = LinearDiscriminantAnalysis(n _ components=2)
X_r2 = lda.fit(X, y).transform(X)

# Percentage of variance explained for each components
print(
    "explained variance ratio (first two components): %s"
    % str(pca.explained_variance_ratio_)
)

plt.figure()
colors = ["Red", "Green", "Blue"]

for color, i, target _ name in zip(colors, [0, 1, 2], target _ names):
    plt.scatter(
        X_r[y == i, 0], X_r[y == i, 1], color=color,
alpha=0.8,label=target_name
    )
plt.legend(loc="best", shadow=False, scatterpoints=1)
plt.title("PCA of IRIS dataset")

plt.figure()
for color, i, target_name in zip(colors, [0, 1, 2], target_names):
    plt.scatter(
        X_r2[y == i, 0], X_r2[y == i, 1], alpha=0.8, color=color,
label=target_name
    )
plt.legend(loc="best", shadow=False, scatterpoints=1)
plt.title("LDA of IRIS dataset")

plt.show()
```

3.6 CONCLUSION

The chapter's exploration into feature extraction techniques using Python—Principal Components Analysis (PCA), Kernel PCA (KPCA), Independent Component Analysis (ICA), and Linear Discriminant Analysis (LDA)—has been an enlightening journey, revealing the significance of refining data in machine learning. Through Python implementations, PCA effectively reduces dimensions by capturing data variance, simplifying complexity while retaining crucial information. KPCA extends this ability by handling nonlinear data structures adeptly. Additionally, ICA highlights the extraction of statistically independent components, unveiling latent factors within the data. Meanwhile, LDA's Python demonstrations emphasize its role in enhancing supervised learning by optimizing class separability. These Python-based explorations illustrate the practicality and effectiveness of these feature extraction techniques across various domains. The chapter underscores these methods' adaptability in diverse fields like image processing, signal analysis, and text mining. Ultimately, these techniques empower machine learning models to recognize significant patterns, advancing their accuracy and adaptability in different data-driven tasks.

REFERENCES

[1] F. Shahzad, Z. Huang, and W. H. Memon, "Process Monitoring Using Kernel PCA and Kernel Density Estimation-Based SSGLR Method for Nonlinear Fault Detection," *Applied Science*, vol. 12, p. 2981, 2022.

[2] L. Asiedu, A. Adebanji, F. Oduro, and F. Mettle, "Statistical Assessment of PCA/SVD and FFT-PCA/SVD on Variable Facial Expressions," *British Journal of Mathematics & Computer Science*, vol. 12, pp. 1–23, 2016.

[3] M. Journ and P. Richt, "Generalized Power Method for Sparse Principal Component Analysis," *Journal of Machine Learning Research*, vol. 11, pp. 517–553, 2010.

[4] N. Kumar, S. Singh, and A. Kumar, "Random Permutation Principal Component Analysis for Cancelable Biometric Recognition," *Applied Intelligence*, vol. 48, pp. 2824–2836, 2018.

[5] E. Barshan, A. Ghodsi, Z. Azimifar, and M. Zolghadri Jahromi, "Supervised Principal Component Analysis: Visualization, Classification and Regression on Subspaces and Submanifolds," *Pattern Recognition*, vol. 44, pp. 1357–1371, 2011.

[6] A. K. Uysal, "On Two-Stage Feature Selection Methods for Text Classification," *IEEE Access*, vol. 6, pp. 43233–43251, 2018.

[7] A. Karami, "Application of Fuzzy Clustering for Text Data Dimensionality Reduction" *International Journal of Knowledge Engineering and Data Mining*, vol. 6, p. 289, 2019.

[8] H. Jégou and O. Chum, "Negative Evidences and Co-Occurrences in Image Retrieval: The Benefit of PCA and Whitening." In: A. Fitzgibbon, S. Lazebnik, P. Perona, Y. Sato, and C. Schmid, Eds., *Lecture Notes in Computer Science*, Springer, Berlin, pp. 774–787, 2012.

[9] G. Rajitha and K. U. Raju, "PCA-ICA Based Acoustic Ambient Extraction," *International Journal of Scientific Research in Computer Science, Engineering and Information Technology*, vol. 3, pp. 51–59, 2018.

[10] S. Dong, R. Hu, W. Tu, X. Zheng, J. Jiang, and S. Wang, "Enhanced Principal Component Using Polar Coordinate PCA for Stereo Audio Coding," in: *2012 IEEE International Conference on Multimedia and Expo*, Melbourne, Jul 9–13, 2012, pp. 628–633.

[11] T. Bouwmans, S. Javed, H. Zhang, Z. Lin, and R. Otazo, "On the Applications of Robust PCA in Image and Video Processing," *Proceedings of the IEEE*, vol. 106, pp. 1427–1457, 2018.

[12] J. Arunnehru and M. K. Geetha "Motion Intensity Code for Action Recognition in Video Using PCA and SVM." In: R. Prasath and T. Kathirvalavakumar, Eds., *Lecture Notes in Computer Science*, Springer: Cham, pp. 70–81, 2013.

[13] W. Li, M. Han and S. Feng, "Multivariate Chaotic Time Series Prediction: Broad Learning System Based on Sparse PCA." in: T. Gedeon, K. W. Wong, M. Lee, and C. Z. Xu, Eds., *International Conference on Neural Information Processing*, Springer International Publishing, Berlin, pp. 56–66, 2018.

[14] S. Divya and G. Padmavathi, "A Novel Method for Detection of Internet Worm Malcodes Using Principal Component Analysis and Multiclass Support Vector Machine," *International Journal of Security and Its Applications*, vol. 8, pp. 391–402, 2014.

[15] H. Shin, H. Jeong, J. Park, S. Hong, and Y. Choi "Correlation between Cancerous Exosomes and Protein Markers Based on Surface-Enhanced Raman Spectroscopy (SERS) and Principal Component Analysis (PCA)," *ACS Sensors*, vol. 3, pp. 2637–2643, 2018.

[16] R. Osadchy, *Kernel PCA—Unsupervised Learning 2011*, PPT Presentation, p. 26, 2011.

[17] X. F. Liu and C. Yang, "Greedy Kernel PCA for Training Data Reduction and Nonlinear Feature Extraction in Classification." MIPPR 2009: Automatic Target Recognition and Image Analysis, 7495, Article ID: 749530, 2009.

[18] Y. Washizawa, "Subset Kernel Principal Component Analysis", in: *2009 IEEE International Workshop on Machine Learning for Signal Processing*, Grenoble, September 1–4, 2009, pp. 1–6.

[19] M. Debruyne and T. Verdonck, "Robust Kernel Principal Component Analysis and Classification," *Advances in Data Analysis and Classification*, vol. 4, pp. 151–167, 2010.

[20] J. Chen, G. Wang, and G. B. Giannakis, "Nonlinear Dimensionality Reduction for Discriminative Analytics of Multiple Datasets," *IEEE Transactions on Signal Processing*, vol. 67, pp. 740–752, 2019.

[21] K. I. Kim, M. O. Franz, and B. Sch, Image Modeling Based on Kernel Principal Component Analysis," *IEEE Transactions on Pattern Analysis and Machine Intelligence*, vol. 9, pp. 1–17, 2014.

[22] C. Leitner, F. Pernkopf, and G. Kubin, "Kernel PCA for Speech Enhancement. NTERSPEECH 2011", in: *12th Annual Conference of the International Speech Communication Association*, Florence, August 27–31, 2011, pp. 1221–1224.

[23] C. Leitner and F. Pernkopf, "The Pre-Image Problem and Kernel PCA for Speech Enhancement," in: C. M. Travieso-González and J. B. Alonso-Hernández, Eds., *Advances in Nonlinear Speech Processing*, Lecture Notes in Computer Science, vol. 7015, Springer, Berlin, Heidelberg, 2011.

[24] C. Fei and H. Chongzhao, "Time Series Forecasting Based on Wavelet KPCA and Support Vector Machine," in: *2007 IEEE International Conference on Automation and Logistics*, Jinan, August 18–21, 2007, pp. 1487–1491.

[25] J. Ni, H. Ma, and L. Ren, "A Time-Series Forecasting Approach Based on KPCA-LSSVM for Lake Water Pollution," in: *2012 9th International Conference on Fuzzy Systems and Knowledge Discovery*, Chongqing, May, 29–31 2012, pp. 1044–1048.

[26] H. Hoffmann, "Kernel PCA for Novelty Detection," *Pattern Recognition*, vol. 40, pp. 863–874, 2007.

[27] Y. Fan, H. Wang, X. Zhao, Q. Yang, and Y. Liang, "Short-Term Load Forecasting of Distributed Energy System Based on Kernel Principal Component Analysis and KELM Optimized by Fireworks Algorithm," *Applied Science*, vol. 11, p. 12014, 2021.

[28] A. Hyvärinen and E. Oja, "A Fast Fixed-Point Algorithm for Independent Component Analysis," *Neural Computation*, vol 9, pp. 1483–1492, 1997.

[29] S.-I. Amari, A. Cichocki, and H. H. Yang, "A New Learning Algorithm for Blind Source Separation," in: M. Mozer, Ed., *Advances in Neural Information Processing System*, Morgan Kaufmann Publishers, Burlington, MA, pp. 757–763, 1996.

[30] X. S. He, F. He, and A.-L. He, "Super-Gaussian BSS Using Fast-ICA with Chebyshev-Pade Approximant," *Circuits, Systems, and Signal Processing*, vol. 37, pp. 305–341, 2018.

[31] A. Akkalkotkar and K. S. Brown, "An Algorithm for Separation of Mixed Sparse and Gaussian Sources," *PLoS ONE*, vol. 12, p. e0175775, 2017.

[32] T. Radüntz, J. Scouten, O. Hochmuth, and B. Meffert, "Automated EEG Artifact Elimination by Applying Machine Learning Algorithms to ICA-Based Features," *Journal of Neural Engineering*, vol. 14, Article ID: 046004, 2017.

[33] J. Rahmanishamsi, A. Dolati, and M. R. Aghabozorgi, "A Copula Based ICA Algorithm and Its Application to Time Series Clustering," *Journal of Classification*, vol. 35, pp. 230–249, 2018.

[34] M. F. Glasser, T. S. Coalson, J. D. Bijsterbosch, S. J. Harrison, M. P. Harms, A. Anticevic, and S. M. Smith, "Using temporal ICA to Selectively Remove Global Noise While Preserving Global Signal in Functional MRI Data," *NeuroImage*, vol. 181, pp. 692–717, 2018.

[35] H. Ince and T. B. Trafalis, "A Hybrid Forecasting Model for Stock Market Prediction," *Economic Computation and Economic Cybernetics Studies and Research*, vol. 51, pp. 263–280, 2017.

[36] G. Salimi-Khorshidi, G. Douaud, C. F. Beckmann, M. F. Glasser, L. Griffanti, and S. M. Smith, "Automatic Denoising of Functional MRI Data: Combining independent Component Analysis and Hierarchical Fusion of Classifiers," *NeuroImage*, vol. 90, pp. 449–468, 2014.

[37] N. Abrahamsen and P. Rigollet, Sparse Gaussian ICA. 1–27, 2018, http://arxiv.org/abs/1804.00408

[38] P. Ablin, J. F. Cardoso, and A. Gramfort, "Faster ICA Under Orthogonal Constraint," in: *2018 IEEE International Conference on Acoustics, Speech and Signal Processing (ICASSP)*, Calgary, April 15–20, 2018, pp. 4464–4468.

[39] E. Bingham, J. Kuusisto, and K. Lagus, "ICA and SOM in Text Document Analysis. SIGIR Forum (ACM Special Interest Group on Information Retrieval)," August 2002, pp. 361–362.

[40] T. H. Le, "Applying Artificial Neural Networks for Face Recognition," *Advances in Artificial Neural Systems*, vol. 2011, pp. 1–16, 2011.

[41] M. Saimurugan and K. I. Ramachandran, "A Comparative Study of Sound and Vibration Signals in Detection of Rotating Machine Faults Using Support Vector Machine and Independent Component Analysis," *International Journal of Data Analysis Techniques and Strategies*, vol. 7, pp. 188–204, 2015.

[42] C. Agurto, S. Barriga, M. Burge, and P. Soliz, "Characterization of Diabetic Peripheral Neuropathy in Infrared Video Sequences Using Independent Component Analysis," in: *2015 IEEE 25th International Workshop on Machine Learning for Signal Processing (MLSP)*, Boston, MA, September 17–20, 2015, pp. 1–6.

[43] H. Grigoryan, "A Stock Market Prediction Method Based on Support Vector Machines (SVM) and Independent Component Analysis (ICA)," *Database Systems Journal*, vol. 7, pp. 12–21, 2016.

[44] R. C. Welsh, L. M. Jelsone-Swain, and B. R. Foerster, "The Utility of Independent Component Analysis and Machine Learning in the Identification of the Amyotrophic Lateral Sclerosis Diseased Brain," *Frontiers in Human Neuroscience*, vol. 7, pp. 1–9, 2013.

[45] E. M. Fisher, "Linear Discriminant Analysis," *Statistics & Discrete Methods of Data Sciences*, vol. 392, pp. 1–5, 1936.

[46] F. Pan, G. Song, X. Gan, and Q. Gu, "Consistent Feature Selection and Its Application to Face Recognition," *Journal of Intelligent Information Systems*, vol. 43, pp. 307–321, 2014.

[47] A. Sharma and K. K. Paliwal, "A New Perspective to Null Linear Discriminant Analysis Method and Its Fast Implementation Using Random Matrix Multiplication with Scatter Matrices," *Pattern Recognition*, vol. 45, pp. 2205–2213, 2012.

[48] P. N. Belhumeur, J. P. Hespanha, and D. J. Kriegman, "Eigenfaces vs. Fisherfaces: Recognition Using Class Specific Linear Projection," *IEEE Transactions on Pattern Analysis and Machine Intelligence*, vol. 19, pp. 711–720, 1997.

[49] W. Yang and H. Wu, "Regularized Complete Linear Discriminant Analysis," *Neurocomputing*, vol. 137, pp. 185–191, 2014.

[50] K. K. Paliwal and A. Sharma, "Improved Pseudoinverse Linear Discriminant Analysis Method for Dimensionality Reduction," *International Journal of Pattern Recognition and Artificial Intelligence*, vol. 26, pp. 1–9, 2012.

[51] R. Ran, B. Fang, X. Wu, and S. Zhang, "A Simple and Effective Generalization of exponential Matrix Discriminant Analysis and Its Application to Face Recognition," *IEICE Transactions on Information and Systems*, vol. E101D, pp. 265–268, 2018.

[52] S. Wang, J. Lu, X. Gu, H. Du, and J. Yang, "Semi-Supervised Linear Discriminant Analysis for Dimension Reduction and Classification," *Pattern Recognition*, vol. 57, pp. 179–189, 2016.

[53] M. Kedadouche, Z. Liu, and M. Thomas, "Bearing Fault Feature Extraction Using Autoregressive Coefficients, Linear Discriminant Analysis and Support Vector Machine under Variable Operating Conditions," *Applied Condition Monitoring*, vol. 9, pp. 339–352, 2018.

[54] H. Xiong, W. Cheng, W. Hu, J. Bian, and Z. Guo, "FWDA: A Fast Wishart Discriminant Analysis with its Application to Electronic Health Records Data Classification," *CoRR*, vol. 1704, no. 1, pp. 1–15, 2017.

[55] L. Wu, C. H. Shen, and A. van den Hengel, "Deep Linear Discriminant Analysis on Fisher Networks: A Hybrid Architecture for Person Re-Identification," *Pattern Recognition*, vol. 65, pp. 238–250, 2017.

[56] A. Krasoulis, K. Nazarpour, and S. Vijayakumar, "Use of Regularized Discriminant Analysis Improves Myoelectric Hand Movement Classification," in: *2017 8th International IEEE/EMBS Conference on Neural Engineering (NER)*, Shanghai, May 25–28, 2017, pp. 395–398.

[57] V. Jusas and S. G. Samuvel "Classification of Motor Imagery Using a Combination of User-Specific Band and Subject-Specific Band for Brain-Computer Interface," *Applied Sciences (Switzerland)*, vol. 9, pp. 1–17, 2019.

[58] S. R. Wilson, M. E. Close, and P. Abraham, "Applying Linear Discriminant Analysis to Predict Groundwater Redox Conditions Conducive to Denitrification," *Journal of Hydrology*, vol. 556, pp. 611–624, 2018.

[59] S. S. Suhas, "Face Recognition Using Principal Component Analysis and Linear Discriminant Analysis on Holistic Approach in Facial Images Database," *IOSR Journal of Engineering*, vol. 2, pp. 15–23, 2012.

[60] Z. Wang, Q. Ruan, and G. An, "Facial expression Recognition Based on Tensor Local Linear Discriminant Analysis," in: *2012 IEEE 11th International Conference on Signal Processing*, Beijing, October 21–25, 2012, pp. 1226–1229.

[61] Y. Sharma, T. Pl, N. Hammerla, S. Mellor, R. Mcnaney, P. Olivier, and I. Essa, "Automated Surgical Osats Prediction from Videos," in: *2014 IEEE 11th International Symposium on Biomedical Imaging (ISBI)*, Beijing, April 29–May 2, 2014, pp. 461–464.

[62] M. H. Siddiqi, R. Ali, M. S. Rana, E. K. Hong, E. S. Kim, and S. Lee, "Video-Based Human Activity Recognition Using Multilevel Wavelet Decomposition and Stepwise Linear Discriminant Analysis," *Sensors (Switzerland)*, vol. 14, pp. 6370–6392, 2014.

[63] E. A. Maharaj and A. M. Alonso, "Discriminant Analysis of Multivariate Time Series: Application to Diagnosis Based on ECG Signals," *Computational Statistics and Data Analysis*, vol. 70, pp. 67–87, 2014.

[64] U. Sakarya and C. Demirpolat, "SAR Image Time-Series Analysis Framework Using Morphological Operators and Global and Local Information-Based Linear Discriminant Analysis," *Turkish Journal of Electrical Engineering and Computer Sciences*, vol. 26, pp. 2958–2966, 2018.

[65] R. Varatharajan, G. Manogaran, and M. K. Priyan, "A Big Data Classification Approach Using LDA with an Enhanced SVM Method for ECG Signals in Cloud Computing," *Multimedia Tools and Applications*, vol. 77, pp. 10195–10215, 2018.

[66] B. V. Dasarathy, "Nosing Around the Neighborhood: A New System Structure and Classification Rule for Recognition in Partially Exposed Environments," *IEEE Transactions on Pattern Analysis and Machine Intelligence*, vol. PAMI-2, no. 1, pp. 67–71, 1980.

[67] F. Pedregosa, G. Varoquaux, A. Gramfort, V. Michel, B. Thirion, O. Grisel, M. Blondel, P. Prettenhofer, R. Weiss, V. Dubourg, J. Verplas, A. Passos, D. Cournapeau, M. Brucher, M. Perrot, and E. Duchesnay, "Scikit-learn: Machine Learning in Python," *Journal of Machine Learning Research*, vol. 12, pp. 2825–2830, 2011.

## CHAPTER 4

Deep Learning and XAI with Python

4.1 INTRODUCTION

The evolution of artificial intelligence (AI) technology is ushering in fresh opportunities across various practical applications [1–100]. Within the diverse landscape of artificial intelligence research, machine learning emerges as a crucial domain, significantly contributing to the development of intelligent systems. Over the last four decades, machine learning, intense learning, has made substantial strides, instigating transformative shifts across multiple research domains. In contrast to initial shallow machine learning tools like Support Vector Machines, AdaBoost, random forests, and K-nearest neighbors, deep learning methods have garnered considerable attention from pattern recognition researchers in recent times. Convolutional Neural Networks (CNN), renowned for their robust discriminative power, have gained popularity, especially in image processing. CNN, a subset of deep learning, involves feature extractions and convolutional stacks to construct a progressive hierarchy of abstract features. Components like convolution, pooling, tangent squashing, rectifier, and normalization form the essential building blocks of a CNN. While CNN-based deep learning efficiently recognizes patterns in visual environments, such as large-scale object detection in images, its application is more geared toward single-image pattern recognition than temporal information decoding. Recurrent Neural Networks (RNNs), particularly the Long Short-Term Memory (LSTM) network, stand out for their capability in time-sequential event analysis, providing superior discriminative power. Despite the effectiveness of these deep learning approaches in their respective fields, their sensitivity to noise poses challenges, potentially impacting system accuracy. TensorFlow, an open-source tool by Google, stands out as a widely utilized platform among deep learning tools for diverse event modelling tasks, including prediction-related activities in pattern recognition. Neural Structured Learning (NSL), another noteworthy open-source framework, represents a cutting-edge deep learning algorithm dedicated to learning events within data. NSL finds applications in

DOI: 10.1201/9781003425908-4

constructing robust models across various research fields, such as computer vision and natural language processing. It leverages structured signals related to feature inputs, employing a neural graph learning approach that depends on graphs and structured data. NSL also extends its capabilities to generalize essential adversarial learning, utilizing structured data with rich relational information among samples. As the AI community strives to meet expectations promptly, it faces a significant hurdle in the explainability problem (XAI), emerging alongside recent AI successes. The need for explainability becomes crucial in the practical application of current AI models. Figure 4.1 shows a wide range of domains related to machine learning, including shallow, deep, and explainable machine learning.

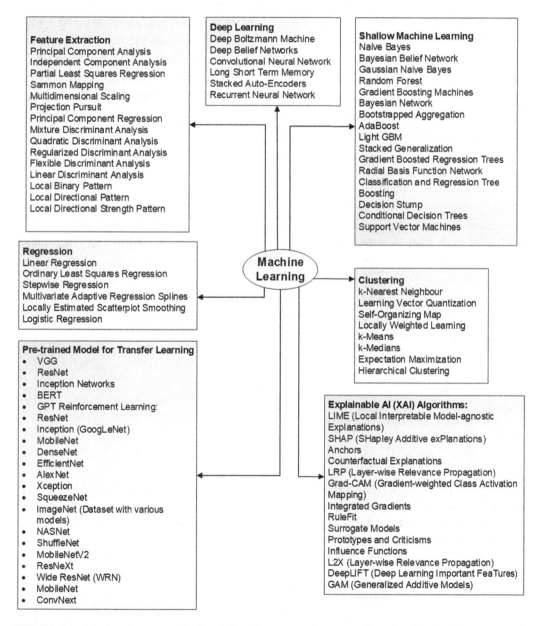

FIGURE 4.1   Machine learning and related algorithms.

With XAI evolving as a core focus of future research within the AI community, a comprehensive examination of its existing contributions is essential, directing attention toward future prospects. Consequently, AI researchers should embrace the concept of trustworthy AI, delving into XAI for large-scale implementations of AI techniques in organizations, with a primary focus on explainability, fairness, and accountability. The recent successes of machine learning models owe much to efficient deep learning algorithms operating within vast parametric spaces, comprising hundreds of layers and millions of parameters. This complex nature transforms deep learning models into intricate black-box systems. Consequently, black-box machine learning models witness increased adoption daily, driving a surge in transparency demands within various contexts. Stakeholders in the AI industry insist on transparency to mitigate risks associated with unjustifiable and illegitimate AI decisions. Therefore, elucidating the output of a model becomes imperative. This chapter aims to articulate diverse machine learning techniques, encompassing both shallow and deep approaches, alongside a dedicated exploration of XAI. The subsequent sections will explore various facets of machine learning and XAI, presenting a comprehensive overview.

4.2 NON-DEEP MACHINE LEARNING

As far as conventional feature analysis is concerned, this involves extracting features from textures, contours, intensity, and various statistical factors, which are then applied to machine learning classifiers such as Decision Trees, Support Vector Machines (SVM), AdaBoost, and deep learning to detect the underlying events within the data. Deep learning generally uses overfitting to solve problems when the data is low in dimension. Considering the fact that shallow learning algorithms can achieve the same degree of accuracy as deep learning, such algorithms are appropriate in this situation [1–66]. The following shallow machine learning will be explained using *iris dataset* available in *sklearn*. Let's see what the dataset looks like.

```
import numpy as np
import pandas as pd
import seaborn as sns
from sklearn import datasets

iris = datasets.load _iris()
df = pd.DataFrame(iris.data, columns=iris.feature_names)
# sklearn provides the iris species as integer values since this
is required for classification
# here we're just adding a column with the species names to the
dataframe for visualisation
df['species'] = np.array([iris.target_names[i] for i in iris.
target])
sns.pairplot(df, hue='species')
```

The code generates following pair plot figure:

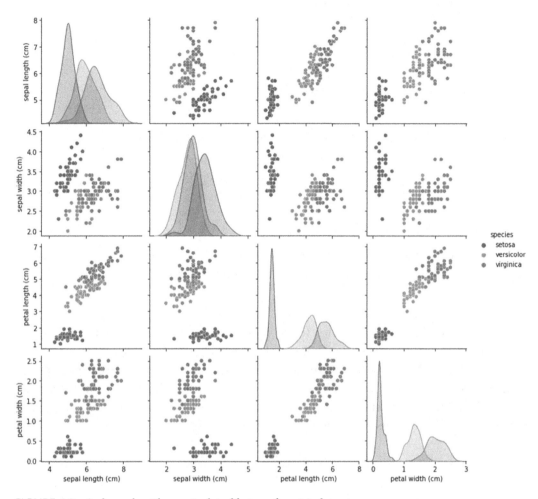

FIGURE 4.2   Seaborn algorithms pair plot of features from iris dataset.

We can notice that iris-setosa is easily identifiable by petal length and petal width, while the other two species are much more difficult to distinguish. Figure 4.2 shows seaborn algorithms pair plot of features from the iris dataset.

4.2.1 Support Vector Machines

To address classification and regression challenges, Support Vector Machines (SVM) formulate one or more high-dimensional hyperplanes. SVM facilitates the creation of an optimized hyperplane situated at the maximum distance from the nearest training data sample, leading to an effective separation boundary. The broader the margin, the lower the generalization error of the classifier, and conversely, a narrower margin may result in higher generalization errors. Recognized for their exceptional predictive and generalization capabilities, SVMs stand out as favored models for handling small datasets. Figure 4.3 visually illustrates the data separation between two classes achieved through a linear SVM. This depiction provides a clear representation of how SVM optimally positions the hyperplane to maximize the margin, enhancing its ability to generalize and make accurate predictions, particularly beneficial in scenarios involving limited data.

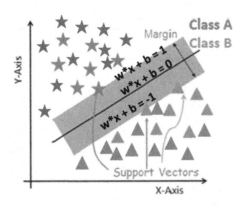

FIGURE 4.3   A linear SVM example.

A large margin classifier between the two classes of data can be obtained. Any hyperplane can be mentioned as the set of points x satisfying following:

$$w.x - b = 0$$

where w serves as the normal vector to the hyper-plane. ard margins and soft margins offer options to partition training data, with hard margins applied when the data can be linearly separated without errors. In linear SVM, the objective is to maximize the distance between two classes by selecting two parallel hyperplanes that distinctly differentiate the classes. Rescaling of datasets in this scenario is represented through equations, capturing the separation of each class by a boundary achieved through dataset rescaling.

$$w.x - b = 1$$
$$w.x - b = -1$$

Classifiers are designed so that anything above the boundary in is classified as one class, while anything below the constraint will be classified as another class. Figure 4.4 illustrates the necessity of a nonlinear SVM due to the fact that linear data separation cannot be achieved.

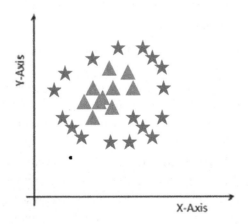

FIGURE 4.4   Necessity of nonlinear SVM.

The advantages of Support Vector Machines are:

- Effective in high dimensional spaces.

- Still effective in cases where the number of dimensions is greater than the number of samples.

- Uses a subset of training points in the decision function (called support vectors), so it is also memory-efficient.

- Versatile: different Kernel functions can be specified for the decision function. Common kernels are provided, but it is also possible to specify custom kernels.

The disadvantages of Support Vector Machines include:

- If the number of features is much greater than the number of samples, avoid overfitting in choosing Kernel functions and regularization term is crucial.

- SVMs do not directly provide probability estimates, these are calculated using an expensive five-fold cross-validation (see Scores and probabilities, below).

```python
import pandas as pd
import numpy as np
from sklearn.svm import SVC
from sklearn.preprocessing import StandardScaler
from sklearn.model_selection import train_test_split
from sklearn.metrics import accuracy_score
from sklearn import datasets

# iris Dataset

iris = datasets.load_iris()
X = iris.data
y = iris.target

# Creating training and test split

X_train, X_test, y_train, y_test = train_test_split(X, y,
test_size=0.3, random_state=1, stratify = y)

# Training a SVM classifier using SVC class
svm = SVC(kernel= 'linear', random_state=1, C=0.1)
svm.fit(X_train, y_train)

# Model performance

y_pred = svm.predict(X_test)
print('Accuracy: %.3f' % accuracy_score(y_test, y_pred))
```

The code generates the following output:
Accuracy: 0.978

4.2.2 Random Forests

As a classifier, the Random Forest is created by randomly choosing the root of each decision tree and generating several Decision Trees. Although Decision Trees are generally straightforward models, their decomposable nature can be a drawback. They follow hierarchical structures for decision-making, which is beneficial for classification problems. The use of Decision Trees has been closely linked to decision-making contexts due to their complexity and interpretability. Currently, tree ensembles are considered the most accurate models in use. These ensembles aim to mitigate overfitting issues associated with individual Decision Trees in machine learning. To address this problem, tree ensembles combine multiple trees to form a collective prediction. Despite efforts to reduce overfitting, the combination of models results in a complex interpretation of the ensemble results. Figure 4.5 illustrates an example tree from a random forest applied to the iris dataset available in the Python *sklearn* library.

Utilizing an ensemble of Decision Trees to the maximum depth serves as a method for constructing trained Random Forests (RFs). The trees within the forest undergo training by employing randomly selected features from a given dataset. Each split node within the tree consists of a feature and a threshold. For classifying a data point d in the data sample S, repeated evaluations of following probabilistic equation are carried out by branching left or right based on a comparison with the threshold. A probability distribution is stored at the leaf node of the tree, $P_T(l|S, x)$ over class l, and subsequently all N distributions are averaged together to give the final classification as follows:

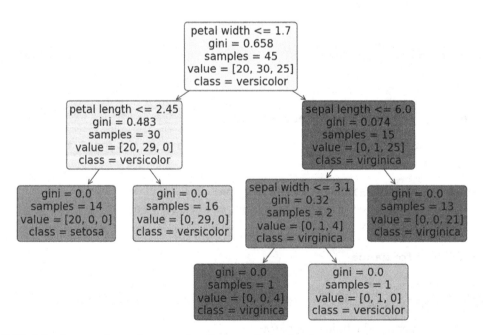

FIGURE 4.5   An example tree from a random forest applied on iris dataset.

$$P(d \mid S, x) = \frac{1}{N} \sum_{T=1}^{N} P_T(l \mid S, x)$$

We can include following code at the end of the last code of SVM and see the results for the same data.

```
# Training a Randomforest classifier using SVC class
from sklearn.ensemble import RandomForestClassifier

#Create a Randomforest Classifier
clf= RandomForestClassifier(n_estimators=100, oob_score=True,
random_state=123456)
#Train the model using the training sets Randomforest Classifier
clf.fit(X_train,y_train)

# Model performance
y_pred = clf.predict(X_test)
print('Accuracy: %.3f' % accuracy_score(y_test, y_pred))
```

The code generates the following output:
Accuracy: 0.956

To see the tree and decisions taken by the algorithm, we can use following:

```
import matplotlib.pyplot as plt
fn=['sepal length', 'sepal width', 'petal length', 'petal width']
cn=['setosa', 'versicolor','virginica']

import matplotlib.pyplot as plt
from sklearn.tree import plot_tree

fig = plt.figure(figsize=(15, 10))
plot_tree(rf.estimators_[0],
    feature_names=fn,
    class_names=cn,
    filled=True, impurity=True,
    rounded=True)
```

4.2.3 AdaBoost and Gradient Boosting

Among the most commonly used ensemble classifiers, the boosting approach [41–61] can be utilized to improve classification by using shallow learning techniques. AdaBoost is one of the most successful boosting classifiers. Its objective is to combine weak learners into a strong one to improve the performance of a learning model by combining weak learners into a strong one. AdaBoost is a method of training samples on poor-performing classifiers by setting weights on them in each iteration. A new weak learning classifier is obtained for the newly weighted data by increasing the weights for misclassified samples and reducing the weights for correctly classified samples. It is repeated until all samples have been correctly classified or until the maximum number of iterations is reached.

```
# Training an AdaBoost classifier using SVC class
from sklearn.ensemble import AdaBoostClassifier

#Create an AdaBoost Classifier
clf=AdaBoostClassifier()

#Train the model using the AdaBoost Classifier
clf.fit(X_train_std,y_train)

# Model performance
y_pred = clf.predict(X_test)
print('Accuracy: %.3f' % accuracy_score(y_test, y_pred))
```

The code generates the following output:
Accuracy: 0.911

Utilizing multiple weak classifiers to enhance the performance of such classifiers character-izes Gradient Boosting. The residuals from one weak classifier are employed as input for another weak classifier, with Decision Trees often serving as these weak classifiers to elevate classification performance. Monitoring the gradient of learning for the connected weak clas-sifiers is accomplished through a learning rate. The method of appreciating negative gradi-ents is the core principle behind Gradient Boosting, leading to its nomenclature. The combination of weak learners results in the development of both a learning procedure and a model to train data. The construction of new base-learners defines enhancements, and GBM parameters are established through a parametric study. Further fine-tuning of the algorithms is then conducted to explore whether additional parameters can enhance their performance. A model with size M can be considered as a linear combination of M+1 base models as

$$D_M(x) = \sum_{i=0}^{M} \beta_i h_i(x)$$

where D_M represents the ith base model and h_i consists of that model's weight.

```
# Training a GradientBoosting classifier using SVC class
from sklearn.ensemble import GradientBoostingClassifier

#Create a Randomforest Classifier
clf=GradientBoostingClassifier(n_estimators=300,learning_
rate=0.05,random_state=100,max_features=4)

#Train the model using the GradientBoosting classifier
clf.fit(X_train_std,y_train)
```

```
# Model performance
y_pred = clf.predict(X_test_std)
print('Accuracy: %.3f' % accuracy_score(y_test, y_pred))
```

The code generates the following output:
Accuracy: 0.956

In addition to solving regression problems, Light GBM can also be used to solve classification problems. The researchers stated that when the models were developed based on Light GBM, it is a gradient lifting framework, which is based-on Decision Tree algorithm, and the parameters suitable for Light GBM were selected by parametric studies. To install Light GBM, we can use *pip install lightgbm*. The following code segment is to use Light GBM.

```
# Training a lightgbm classifier using SVC class
from lightgbm import LGBMClassifier

#Create a lightgbm Classifier
clf=LGBMClassifier()

#Train the model using the lightgbm Classifier
clf.fit(X_train,y_train)

# Model performance
y_pred = clf.predict(X_test)
print('Accuracy: %.3f' % accuracy_score(y_test, y_pred))
```

The code generates the following output:
Accuracy: 0.978

4.2.4 Nearest Neighbors

With Nearest Neighbors (NN) classification algorithms, the problems are dealt with in an extremely straightforward manner. It predicts the class of a sample based on the voting results of its K-nearest neighbors. The neighborhood is determined by the distance between samples, which represents the sample distance. As a replacement for the voting methods in regression problems, a combination of the target values associated with the K-nearest neighbors is used [62–65]. A very interesting matter is that this approach of prediction resembles the experience-based human decision-making in which a decision is made in accordance with the results of previous similar cases. Calculate the Euclidean distance from all training data points as follows:

$$d = \sqrt{\sum_{i=1}^{n} (x_i - y_i)^2}.$$

Based on which, *k*-nearest neighbors are found to assign a class containing the maximum number of nearest neighbors. Let's add the following code in addition to the previous code and see the result.

```
from sklearn.neighbors import KNeighborsClassifier

# Instantiate learning model (k = 3)
classifier = KNeighborsClassifier(n_neighbors=3)

# Fitting the model
classifier.fit(X_train, y_train)

# Predicting the Test set results
y_pred = classifier.predict(X_test)
print('Accuracy: %.3f' % accuracy_score(y_test, y_pred))
```

The code generates the following output:
Accuracy: 0.956

4.2.5 More Examples

Illustrating the nature of decision boundaries from various classifiers, this example demonstrates the application of several classifiers in scikit-learn on synthetic datasets. It's essential to recognize that the insights gained from these examples might not always directly apply to real-world datasets. The division of data can be more straightforward in high-dimensional spaces, making naive Bayes and linear SVMs potentially better at generalization due to their simplicity compared to other classifiers. In the plots, solid colors represent training points, while testing points are semi-transparent. The lower right corner displays the classification accuracy on the test set. A collection of examples has been generated using the scikit-learn machine learning library [66]. Figure 4.6 exhibits the application of different shallow machine learning algorithms on three datasets: make moons, make circles, and linearly separable.

```
import numpy as np
import matplotlib.pyplot as plt
from matplotlib.colors import ListedColormap
from sklearn.model_selection import train_test_split
from sklearn.preprocessing import StandardScaler
from sklearn.datasets import make_moons, make_circles,
make_classification
from sklearn.neighbors import KNeighborsClassifier
from sklearn.svm import SVC
from sklearn.tree import DecisionTreeClassifier
from sklearn.ensemble import RandomForestClassifier,
AdaBoostClassifier
from sklearn.naive_bayes import GaussianNB
from sklearn.discriminant_analysis import
LinearDiscriminantAnalysis as LDA
from sklearn.discriminant_analysis import
QuadraticDiscriminantAnalysis as QDA

h = .02 # step size in the mesh
```

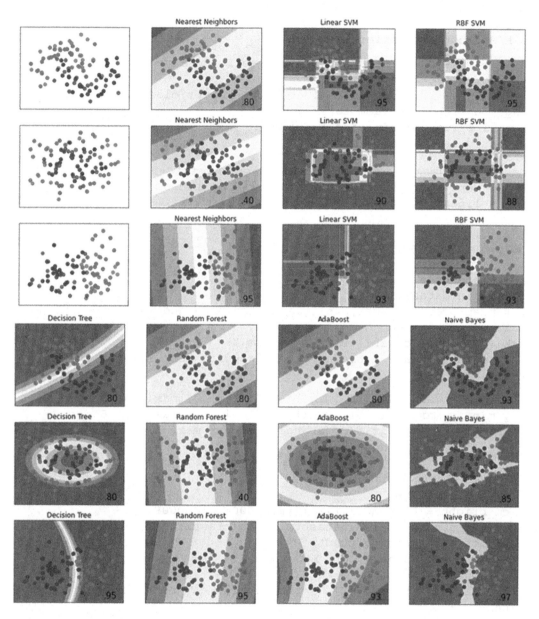

FIGURE 4.6   Different shallow machine learning algorithms applied on three datasets: make moons, make circles, and linearly separable.

```
names = ["Nearest Neighbors", "Linear SVM", "RBF SVM", "Decision Tree",
    "Random Forest", "AdaBoost", "Naive Bayes", "LDA", "QDA"]
classifiers = [
  SVC(kernel="linear", C=0.025),
  RandomForestClassifier(max_depth=5, n_estimators=10,
max_features=2),
  AdaBoostClassifier(),
  GaussianNB(),
  LDA(),
```

```
QDA(),
KNeighborsClassifier(3)]

X, y = make_classification(n_features=2, n_redundant=0,
n_informative=2,
              random_state=1, n_clusters_per_class=1)
rng = np.random.RandomState(2)
X += 2 * rng.uniform(size=X.shape)
linearly_separable = (X, y)

datasets = [make _ moons(noise=0.3, random _ state=0),
      make_circles(noise=0.2, factor=0.5, random_state=1),
      linearly_separable
      ]

figure = plt.figure(figsize=(27, 9))
i = 1
# iterate over datasets
for ds in datasets:
  # preprocess dataset, split into training and test part
  X, y = ds
  X = StandardScaler().fit_transform(X)
  X_train, X_test, y_train, y_test = train_test_split(X, y,
test_size=.4)

  x_min, x_max = X[:, 0].min() - .5, X[:, 0].max() + .5
  y_min, y_max = X[:, 1].min() - .5, X[:, 1].max() + .5
  xx, yy = np.meshgrid(np.arange(x_min, x_max, h),
            np.arange(y_min, y_max, h))

  # just plot the dataset first
  cm = plt.cm.RdBu
  cm_bright = ListedColormap(['#FF0000', '#0000FF'])
  ax = plt.subplot(len(datasets), len(classifiers) + 1, i)
  # Plot the training points
  ax.scatter(X_train[:, 0], X_train[:, 1], c=y_train, cmap=cm_bright)
  # and testing points
  ax.scatter(X_test[:, 0], X_test[:, 1], c=y_test, cmap=cm_bright,
alpha=0.6)
  ax.set_xlim(xx.min(), xx.max())
  ax.set_ylim(yy.min(), yy.max())
  ax.set_xticks(())
  ax.set_yticks(())
  i += 1

  # iterate over classifiers
  for name, clf in zip(names, classifiers):
    ax = plt.subplot(len(datasets), len(classifiers) + 1, i)
    clf.fit(X_train, y_train)
    score = clf.score(X_test, y_test)

    # Plot the decision boundary. For that, we will assign a color
to each
```

```
    # point in the mesh [x_min, m_max]x[y_min, y_max].
    if hasattr(clf, "decision_function"):
      Z = clf.decision_function(np.c_[xx.ravel(), yy.ravel()])
    else:
      Z = clf.predict_proba(np.c_[xx.ravel(), yy.ravel()])[:, 1]

    # Put the result into a color plot
    Z = Z.reshape(xx.shape)
    ax.contourf(xx, yy, Z, cmap=cm, alpha=.8)

    # Plot also the training points
    ax.scatter(X_train[:, 0], X_train[:, 1], c=y_train,
cmap=cm_bright)
    # and testing points
    ax.scatter(X_test[:, 0], X_test[:, 1], c=y_test,
cmap=cm_bright,
          alpha=0.6)

    ax.set_ xlim(xx.min(), xx.max())
    ax.set_ylim(yy.min(), yy.max())
    ax.set_xticks(())
    ax.set_yticks(())
    ax.set_title(name)
    ax.text(xx.max() - .3, yy.min() + .3, ('%.2f' % score).
lstrip('0'),
        size=15, horizontalalignment='right')
    i += 1

figure.subplots _ adjust(left=.02, right=.98)
plt.show()
```

4.3 DEEP MACHINE LEARNING

In the development of automated machine learning models, the learning algorithm strives to identify patterns and relevant relationships within the input data. A shallow learning algorithm typically relies on well-designed features to accomplish its task. Various mechanisms are applied based on this information to construct analytical models through the learning algorithms. For instance, a Decision Tree-based algorithm utilizes the feature space to create a classification model by incrementally partitioning data records into increasingly homogeneous partitions with a tree-like structure. With SVM, a hyper-plane is built between data points of different classes, facilitating their separation. These examples illustrate that there are multiple ways to construct an analytical model, each with its own advantages and disadvantages, depending on the input data and features. Deep learning, known for its automated feature learning capability, can be directly applied to high-dimensional input data for robust model construction, often organized as end-to-end systems. While deep learning algorithms can operate independently, they can also be combined with shallow learning for enhanced performance based on the data's characteristics. In recent decades, various deep learning architectures have emerged, including CNN, RNN, adversarial neural networks, and neural self-learning algorithms [67–108].

4.3.1 Convolutional Neural Networks

Convolutional Neural Networks (CNNs) are inspired by the visual cortex of animals and consist of multiple layers. The initial layers of CNNs are dedicated to extracting features, which are then utilized by subsequent layers to generate higher-level features. To address the dimensionality constraints of these features, the process of pooling is employed, involving repeated convolution and pooling before feeding the results into a fully connected multilayer perceptron. Back-propagation algorithms are employed for recognizing features in the final output layer. The combination of deep processing layers, convolutional networks, pooling algorithms, and a fully connected classification layer has found success in various applications, particularly in image processing and computer vision. CNNs, with their local connectivity and shared weights, enhance accuracy and overall system performance. However, a limitation of convolutional layers is the precise storage of feature positions, which can be addressed by down-sampling to generate a lower-resolution version of the input data while retaining critical structural elements. Down-sampling, achieved by altering the convolution stride or using a pooling layer, helps in handling this issue. Pooling layers, typically added after the convolution layer, can be of two types: maximum and average. To enhance the quality of feature maps, nonlinearity (e.g., ReLU) is often applied before pooling. In summary, a typical CNN layer comprises the input image, convolutional, nonlinearity, and pooling layers. The network undergoes fine-tuning to adjust hyperparameters, providing the convolution layer with distinct characteristics.

$$\text{Convolution}_k^{(i+1)}(m,n) = \text{ReLU}(u),$$

$$\text{ReLU}(u) = \sum_{(g=1)}^{z} \Omega\left(m, \left(n - g + \frac{z+1}{2}\right)\right) W_k^i(g) + \alpha_k^i$$

where $\text{Convolution}_k^{(i+1)}(m,n)$ generates convolution results for (m, n) coordinates of $(i+1)$th layer with kth convolution map. W_k^i is kth *convolution kernel* for ith layer. α_k^i is kth *bias values* for ith layer. Ω is the map of the previous layer and z the size of the kernel. ReLU represents the active function that considers the summation of weights of the previous layer to pass them to the next layer. The second layer is first pooling layer $Pooling_1$. This layer usually down samples the results of $Convolution_1$ to a matrix. In pooling, typically maximum or summation is done using sliding windows in the previous map.

Thus, the pooling results for $(i + 1)$th, kernel k, row x, and column y can be represented as

$$\text{Pooling}_k^{i+1}(x, = \max_{1 \le r \le s}(\text{Convolution}_k^i(x, ((y+s))))$$

where p is the length of the pooling window. Figure 4.7 shows a basic architecture of a sample CNN. First convolution generates a matrix with the size of $32 \times 124 \times 124$ followed by max-pooling that down samples that by 1×2 sliding window and generates a matrix with the size of $32 \times 62 \times 62$. Using similar way, second convolution layer applies 32 convolution kernels and similar to the first pooling layer, 1×2 max-pooling is applied for second as well. At last, the fully connected layer is obtained as

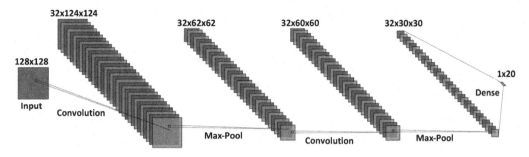

 32x124x124

32x62x62   32x60x60   32x30x30

128x128   1x20

                                                    Dense

Input

Convolution

        Max-Pool   Convolution   Max-Pool

FIGURE 4.7   Basic architecture of a sample CNN.

$$FC_j^{(l+1)} = \text{ReLU}\left(\sum_i x_i^l W_{ij}^{\ l} + \alpha_j^l\right)$$

where $W_{ij}^l \text{w}_{ij}^l$ is a matrix containing weight values from the ith node of the lth layer to the jth node of the $(l+1)$th layer. x_i^l represents the content of ith node at lth layer. Sample code to apply a random CNN model is shown below. Followed by which, Figure 4.8 shows results obtained using the code by applying the CNN model on CIFAR10 dataset. Figure 4.9 shows the train and validation accuracy of the CNN model.

```
import tensorflow as tf

from tensorflow.keras import datasets, layers, models
import matplotlib.pyplot as plt

(train_images, train_labels), (test_images, test_labels) =
datasets.cifar10.load_data()

# Normalize pixel values to be between 0 and 1
train_images, test_images = train_images / 255.0, test_images /
255.0

class_names = ['airplane', 'automobile', 'bird', 'cat', 'deer',
        'dog', 'frog', 'horse', 'ship', 'truck']
#show the sample images
plt.figure(figsize=(10,10))
for i in range(25):
  plt.subplot(5,5,i+1)
  plt.xticks([])
  plt.yticks([])
  plt.grid(False)
  plt.imshow(train_images[i])
  # The CIFAR labels happen to be arrays,
  # which is why you need the extra index
  plt.xlabel(class_names[train_labels[i][0]])
plt.show()
```

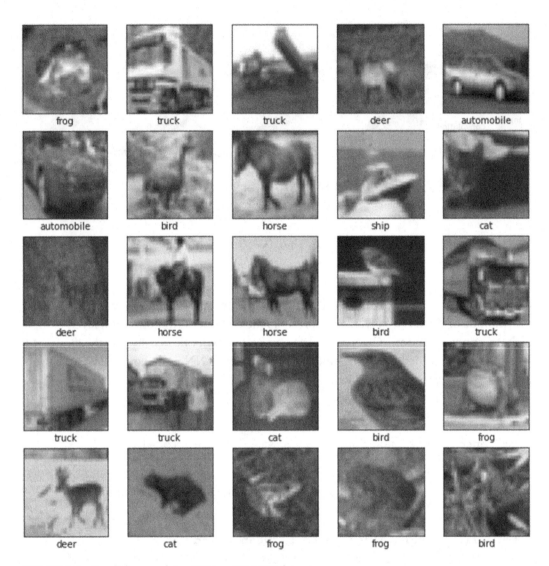

FIGURE 4.8   Result from applying CNN on CIFAR10 dataset.

```
#initialize the cnn model
model = models.Sequential()
model.add(layers.Conv2D(32, (3, 3), activation='relu', input_
shape=(32, 32, 3)))
model.add(layers.MaxPooling2D((2, 2)))
model.add(layers.Conv2D(64, (3, 3), activation='relu'))
model.add(layers.MaxPooling2D((2, 2)))
model.add(layers.Conv2D(64, (3, 3), activation='relu'))
model.add(layers.Flatten())
model.add(layers.Dense(10))
model.summary()
```

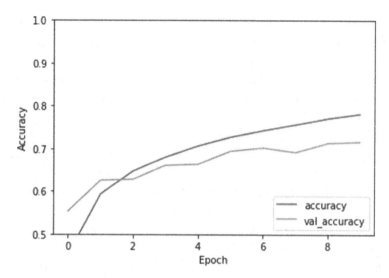

FIGURE 4.9   Train and validation accuracy on applying CNN on CIFAR10 dataset.

```
#compile and train

model.compile(optimizer='adam',
        loss=tf.keras.losses.SparseCategoricalCrossentropy(f
rom_logits=True),
        metrics=['accuracy'])

history = model.fit(train _ images, train _ labels, epochs=10,
          validation_data=(test_images, test_labels))

#training epoch vs accuracy
plt.plot(history.history['accuracy'], label='accuracy')
plt.plot(history.history['val_accuracy'], label = 'val_accuracy')
plt.xlabel('Epoch')
plt.ylabel('Accuracy')
plt.ylim([0.5, 1])
plt.legend(loc='lower right')

#test
test_loss, test_acc = model.evaluate(test_images, test_labels,
verbose=2)
print('The test accuracy is ', test_acc)
```

The output for testing is:
The test accuracy is 0.7157999873161316.

4.3.2 Pre-trained CNN Models

Deep learning methods are typically trained using a greedy approach, particularly effective with large datasets. Initially, the abundance of data posed a significant challenge,
but the landscape changed with the rise of substantial databases and the availability of

hardware-accelerated devices like graphics processing units (GPUs) and cluster computing. This led to an explosion of deep learning research, resulting in a multitude of models. Notably, for large image-related tasks, advancements have been made in training extensive networks and storing CNN-based model weights as pre-trained models. Some prominent models include VGGNet, ResNet, MobileNet, Vision Transformers, Swin Transformers, and the latest ConvNext Transformers.

VGG-16 stands out as a well-known deep convolutional neural network with 16 layers, developed using the extensive ImageNet database. It originated from the Visual Geometry Group at Oxford University. Additionally, VGG-19, a variant with 19 layers, follows the same conceptual foundation as VGG-16. ResNet variants are characterized by their architecture and layer count, with examples like ResNet-18 and ResNet-1202. A notable extension, ResNet V2, incorporates a second non-linearity function as an identity mapping function, building on the foundation of ResNet V1.

The provided code exemplifies the application of different pretrained CNN models on the CIFAR10 dataset, showcasing their outputs in a sample journey.

```
from tensorflow.keras.datasets import cifar10
from tensorflow.keras.preprocessing.image import
ImageDataGenerator
from tensorflow.keras.applications.vgg16 import VGG16
from tensorflow.keras.preprocessing import image
from tensorflow.keras.applications.vgg16 import preprocess_input
from tensorflow.keras.layers import Input, Flatten, Dense
from tensorflow.keras.models import Model
from tensorflow.keras.optimizers import Adam
import numpy as np
from tensorflow.keras import utils
from keras.utils import np_utils


num _ classes = 10
(x_train, y_train), (x_test, y_test) = cifar10.load_data()
y_train = np_utils.to_categorical(y_train, num_classes)
y_test = np_utils.to_categorical(y_test, num_classes)

datagen = ImageDataGenerator()

#Get back the convolutional part of a VGG network trained on
ImageNet
model_vgg16_conv = VGG16(weights='imagenet', include_top=False)
for layer in model_vgg16_conv.layers: layer.trainable=False


#Create your own input format (here 3x200x200)
input = Input(shape=(32,32, 3),name = 'image_input')


#Use the generated model
output_vgg16_conv = model_vgg16_conv(input)
```

```
x = output _ vgg16 _ conv
x = Flatten()(x) # Flatten dimensions to for use in FC layers
x = Dense(256, activation='relu')(x)
x = Dense(num_classes , activation='softmax')(x) # Softmax for multiclass
transfer_model = Model(inputs=input, outputs=x)

learning _ rate= 5e-5
transfer_model.compile(loss="categorical_crossentropy",
optimizer=Adam(lr=learning_rate), metrics=["accuracy"])
history = transfer_model.fit(x_train, y_train, batch_size = 10,
epochs=50, validation_data=(x_test,y_test))
test_loss, test_acc = transfer_model.evaluate(x_test, y_test,
batch_size=10)
print ('The test accuracy is ', test_acc)
```

The output is obtained as bellow.
The test accuracy is 0.51.

Now for VGG19 just replace VGG16 with VGG19 as follows:

```
from tensorflow.keras.applications.vgg19 import VGG19
from tensorflow.keras.applications.vgg19 import preprocess_input

model _ vgg19 _ conv = VGG19(weights='imagenet', include _ top=False)
for layer in model_vgg19_conv.layers: layer.trainable=False
#Use the generated model
output_vgg19_conv = model_vgg19_conv(input)
x = output_vgg19_conv
x = Flatten()(x) # Flatten dimensions to for use in FC layers
x = Dense(256, activation='relu')(x)
x = Dense(num_classes , activation='softmax')(x) # Softmax for
multiclass
transfer_model = Model(inputs=input, outputs=x)

learning _ rate= 5e-5
transfer_model.compile(loss="categorical_crossentropy",
optimizer=Adam(lr=learning_rate), metrics=["accuracy"])
history = transfer_model.fit(x_train, y_train, batch_size = 10,
epochs=50, validation_data=(x_test,y_test))
```

It is important to note that ResNet (ResNet) ensures that the performance of top layers is equally good as the performance of lower layers without vanishing gradients and optimization issues. There are several variations of the ResNet architecture. Each variation employs a different number of layers, but utilizes the same concept. Each variant of the ResNet architecture is referred to as ResNet, and two or more digits are added to the name.

For ResNet50, just replace VGG16 as follows:

```
from tensorflow.keras.applications.resnet50 import ResNet50
from tensorflow.keras.applications.resnet50 import
preprocess_input
```

```
model_resnet50_conv = ResNet50(weights='imagenet',
include_top=False)
for layer in model_resnet50_conv.layers: layer.trainable=False

output _ resnet50 _ conv = model _ resnet50 _ conv(input)
x = output_resnet50_conv
x = Flatten()(x) # Flatten dimensions to for use in FC layers
x = Dense(256, activation='relu')(x)
x = Dense(num_classes , activation='softmax')(x) # Softmax for
multiclass
transfer_model = Model(inputs=input, outputs=x)

learning _ rate= 5e-5
transfer_model.compile(loss="categorical_crossentropy",
optimizer=Adam(lr=learning_rate), metrics=["accuracy"])
history = transfer_model.fit(x_train, y_train, batch_size = 10,
epochs=50, validation_data=(x_test,y_test))
test_loss, test_acc = transfer_model.evaluate(x_test, y_test,
batch_size=10)
print ('The test accuracy is ', test_acc)
```

In comparison to alternative Convolutional Neural Network architectures, Inception stands out for delivering excellent performance while maintaining lower computational costs. The evolution of Inception led to Inceptionv3, a Convolutional Neural Network boasting 48 layers specifically crafted for image analysis and object detection. Initially conceptualized as a Googlenet module, this upgraded version enhances capabilities. Input resizing plays a crucial role in utilizing pretrained models, as the input shape must align with the model. The application of Inception V3 involves:

```
import tensorflow as tf
from tensorflow.keras.layers import Reshape, Dropout, Dense,
Multiply, Dot, Concatenate, Embedding
from tensorflow.keras.applications.inception_v3 import
InceptionV3, preprocess_input
from tensorflow.keras import models
from tensorflow.keras import layers
from tensorflow.keras import optimizers
from keras.utils import np_utils
from keras.models import load_model
from keras.datasets import cifar10

conv _ base = InceptionV3(weights='imagenet', include _ top=False,
input _ shape=(256, 256, 3))

(x _ train, y _ train), (x _ test, y _ test) = cifar10.load _ data()

x _ train = x _ train / 255.0
x_test = x_test / 255.0
```

```
y_train = np_utils.to_categorical(y_train, 10)
y_test = np_utils.to_categorical(y_test, 10)

transfer_model = models.Sequential()
transfer_model.add(layers.UpSampling2D((2,2)))        ## UpSampling
increase the row and column of the data. Sometimes if we have less
data so we can try to increase the data in this way.
transfer_model.add(layers.UpSampling2D((2,2)))
transfer_model.add(layers.UpSampling2D((2,2)))
transfer_model.add(conv_base)               ## conv_base is the
inception network.We are keeping it here.
transfer_model.add(layers.Flatten())
transfer_model.add(layers.Dense(128, activation='relu' ))
transfer_model.add(layers.Dropout(0.5))
transfer_model.add(layers.BatchNormalization())
transfer_model.add(layers.Dense(64, activation='relu'))
transfer_model.add(layers.Dropout(0.5))
transfer_model.add(layers.BatchNormalization())
transfer_model.add(layers.Dense(10, activation='softmax'))
transfer_model.compile(optimizer='adam', loss='categorical_
crossentropy', metrics=['acc'])

history = transfer_model.fit(x_train, y_train, steps_per_
epoch=10, epochs=3, batch_size=32, validation_data=(x_test,
y_test))

test_loss, test_acc = transfer_model.evaluate(x_test, y_test,
batch_size=10)
print ('The test accuracy is ', test_acc)
```

It is also possible to extend the Inception architecture with Xception, which replaces Inception modules with depth-wise separable convolutional layers. An Xception model utilizes 36 depth-wise separable (i.e., convolutional) layers on a linear stack. The layers are connected through linear residual connections. There are two types of convolutional layers in Xception: depth-wise convolutional layers and pointwise convolutional layers. As for the architecture, Inception has similar parameters as Xception, but the latter can be optimized for greater performance by efficiently adjusting the parameters of the model. The Xception model can be executed a follows:

```
import tensorflow as tf
from keras import Sequential
from tensorflow.keras.utils import to_categorical
from tensorflow.keras.optimizers import SGD,Adam
from keras.callbacks import ReduceLROnPlateau
from tensorflow.keras.applications import VGG19,Xception
from tensorflow.keras.layers import Input,Flatten,Dense,
BatchNormalization,Activation,Dropout,
GlobalAveragePooling2D,MaxPooling2D,RandomFlip,RandomZoom,
RandomRotation
```

```
(x_train, y_train), (x_val, y_val) = cifar10.load_data()

y_train=to_categorical(y_train)
y_val=to_categorical(y_val)

base_model = Xception(include_top=False, weights='imagenet',
input_shape=(224,224,3), classes=y_train.shape[1])
base_model.trainable = False

data_augmentation = Sequential(
  [RandomFlip("horizontal"),
   RandomRotation(0.1),
   RandomZoom(0.1)]
)
inputs = tf.keras.Input(shape=(32, 32, 3))
x = tf.keras.layers.Lambda(lambda image: tf.image.resize(image,
(224,224)))(inputs)
x = data_augmentation(x)
x = tf.keras.applications.xception.preprocess_input(x)
x = base_model(x, training=False)
x = tf.keras.layers.GlobalAveragePooling2D()(x)
x = tf.keras.layers.Dropout(0.3)(x)
outputs = tf.keras.layers.Dense(10, activation=('softmax'))(x)
transfer_model = tf.keras.Model(inputs, outputs)
transfer_model.compile(optimizer='adam', loss='categorical_
crossentropy', metrics=['acc'])
history = transfer_model.fit(x_train, y_train, steps_per_epoch=10,
epochs=3, batch_size=32, validation_data=(x_test, y_test))

test_loss, test_acc = transfer_model.evaluate(x_test, y_test,
batch_size=10)
print ('The test accuracy is ', test_acc)
```

MobileNet is a lightweight image-classification network that typically performs better than MobileNetV1 being 17 MB with 4.2 million nodes, which is small compared to other networks that have faster performance. These are most useful for mobile applications. MobileNetV2 is a light weight model for image classification which usually outperforms MobileNetV1. Moreover, vision transformers have also received considerable attention from researchers in addition to the previously mentioned models. Using the encoder-decoder architecture, Vision Transformer (ViT) is capable of processing data sequences simultaneously without the need for recurrent networks [109]. Transformer-based models have achieved considerable success in recent years, particularly because of their ability to capture long-range relationships among the sequence elements by using a self-attention mechanism. With ViT, the standard famous Transformer has been extended to image classification problems, which is typically associated with natural language processing. ViT aims to generalize the modalities without integrating any data-specific architecture. The attention mechanism in ViT differs from traditional CNN architectures, which typically apply filters in addition to local receptive fields. ViT integrates information across images and attends to various regions within those images. Therefore, ViT has gained significant popularity as a region-based attention system. ViT model can be coded on CIFAR10 dataset as follows:

```python
import tensorflow as tf
from tensorflow.keras.models import Sequential, Model
from tensorflow.keras.layers import Dense, GlobalAveragePooling2D,
BatchNormalization, Flatten, Dropout, Activation, Input
from tensorflow.keras.utils import to_categorical
from tensorflow.keras.preprocessing.image import
ImageDataGenerator
from tensorflow.keras import optimizers
from tensorflow.keras.callbacks import ReduceLROnPlateau,
EarlyStopping
from tensorflow.keras.datasets import cifar10
from vit_keras import vit, utils
import tensorflow_addons as tfa
from sklearn.model_selection import train_test_split
from sklearn.metrics import accuracy_score
import matplotlib.pyplot as plt
import gc
import numpy as np # linear algebra
import pandas as pd # data processing, CSV file I/O (e.g.
pd.read_csv)


seed = 2022
np.random.seed(seed)
tf.random.set_seed(seed)


(train_data, train_label), (test_data, test_label) = cifar10.
load_data()
train_label = to_categorical(train_label)
test_label = to_categorical(test_label)
train_data = (train_data/255.).astype("float32")
test_data = (test_data/255.).astype("float32")

X_train, X_valid, y_train, y_valid = train_test_split(train_
data, train_label, random_state=seed, shuffle=True)


batch_size = 32
datagen = ImageDataGenerator(rotation_range=15, width_shift_
range=0.2, zoom_range=0.2, horizontal_flip=True)
train_generator = datagen.flow(X_train, y_train,
batch_size=batch_size)


input_shape = (32, 32, 3) #Cifar10 image size
image_size = 256 #size after resizing image
num_classes = 10
inputs = Input(shape=input_shape)
```

```
x = tf.keras.layers.Lambda(lambda image: tf.image.resize(image,
(image_size, image_size)))(inputs) #Resize image to size 224x224
base_model = vit.vit_b16(image_size=image_size,
activation="sigmoid", pretrained=True,include_top=False,
pretrained_top=False)
base_model.trainable = False #Set false for transfer learning

x = base _ model(x)
x = Flatten()(x)
x = BatchNormalization()(x)
x = Dense(32, activation=tfa.activations.gelu)(x)
x = BatchNormalization()(x)
outputs = Dense(num_classes, activation="softmax")(x)
transfer_model = tf.keras.Model(inputs, outputs)
transfer _ model.compile(optimizer=optimizers.SGD(learning _
rate=0.01, momentum=0.9), loss="categorical _ crossentropy",
metrics=["accuracy"])

transfer_model.fit(train_generator,
     steps_per_epoch=200,
     epochs=2,
     validation_data=(X_valid, y_valid),
     )
test_loss, test_acc = transfer_model.evaluate(x_test, y_test,
batch_size=10)
print ('The test accuracy is ', test_acc)
```

The Swin Transformer is a type of vision transformer based on hierarchical feature maps by merging image patches in deeper layers, and then relies on linear computation complexity of input size due to the calculation of self-attention only within each local window of the image [110]. Thus, it can provide a general-purpose backbone for image classification. As an alternative, the previous ViT produces feature maps of a single low resolution with quadratic computation complexity due to estimation of self-attention globally. The SWIN transformers can be applied on CIFAR10 dataset as:

```
import sys
sys.path.append('./Swin-Transformer-TF')

import tensorflow as tf
from tensorflow.keras.models import Sequential, Model
from tensorflow.keras.layers import Dense, GlobalAveragePooling2D,
BatchNormalization, Flatten, Dropout, Activation, Input, Lambda
from tensorflow.keras.utils import to_categorical
from tensorflow.keras.preprocessing.image import
ImageDataGenerator
from tensorflow.keras import optimizers
from tensorflow.keras.callbacks import ReduceLROnPlateau,
EarlyStopping
from tensorflow.keras.datasets import cifar10
```

```
from swintransformer import SwinTransformer
import tensorflow_addons as tfa
from sklearn.model_selection import train_test_split
from sklearn.metrics import accuracy_score
import numpy as np # linear algebra
import pandas as pd # data processing, CSV file I/O (e.g.
pd.read_csv)

seed = 2022
np.random.seed(seed)
tf.random.set_seed(seed)

(train_data, train_label), (test_data, test_label) = cifar10.
load_data()
train_label = to_categorical(train_label)
test_label = to_categorical(test_label)
train_data = (train_data/255.).astype("float32")
test_data = (test_data/255.).astype("float32")

X_train, X_valid, y_train, y_valid = train_test_split(train_
data, train_label, random_state=seed, shuffle=True)

batch_size = 32
datagen = ImageDataGenerator(rotation_range=15, width_shift_
range=0.2, zoom_range=0.2, horizontal_flip=True)
train_generator = datagen.flow(X_train, y_train,
batch_size=batch_size)

input_shape = (32, 32, 3) #Cifar10 image size
image_shape = (224, 224) #size after resizing image
num_classes = 10

inputs = Input(shape=input_shape)
x = Lambda(lambda image: tf.image.resize(image, image_shape))
(inputs) #Resize image to size 224x224
base_model = SwinTransformer("swin_base_224", include_top=False,
pretrained=True)
base_model.trainable = False #Set false for transfer learning
x = base_model(x)
outputs = Dense(num_classes, activation="softmax")(x)
transfer_model = Model(inputs=inputs, outputs=outputs)

transfer_model.compile(optimizer=optimizers.SGD(learning_
rate=0.01, momentum=0.9), loss="categorical_crossentropy",
metrics=["accuracy"])

transfer_model.fit(train_generator,
    steps_per_epoch=200,
    epochs=2,
    validation_data=(X_valid, y_valid),
    )
```

```
test_loss, test_acc = transfer_model.evaluate(x_test, y_test,
batch_size=10)
print ('The test accuracy is ', test_acc)
```

Facebook AI Research has proposed ConvNext as the most robust model so far, particularly for image-related tasks [111]. There are a number of differences between ConvNets and hierarchical vision transformers such as Swin Transformers. They both have similar inductive biases. However, they differ remarkably in their training procedures. As part of ConvNeXt, research has been conducted in order to bridge the gap between the pre-ViT and post-ViT eras for ConvNets. It began with a standard ResNet architecture and then gradually modified it to construct a hierarchical vision Transformer such as Swin. As a result, researchers have developed a family of pure ConvNets known as ConvNeXt. It has been demonstrated that ConvNeXts are superior to Transformers in terms of accuracy, scalability, and robustness in a variety of vision tasks such as ImageNet classification. As a result, ConvNeXt retains the robustness associated with typical ConvNets while at the same time maintaining the fully convolutional nature for both training and testing. In this way, ConvNeXt is extremely easy to implement.

A related code can be seen as executed here https://colab.research.google.com/github/sayakpaul/ConvNeXt-TF/blob/main/notebooks/finetune.ipynb#scrollTo=2e5oy9zmNNID.

4.3.3 Long Short-Term Memory (LSTM)

Data collected from human activity sensors exhibits time-sequential changes, prompting the exploration of machine learning models adept at encoding such temporal information. In this project, Recurrent Neural Networks (RNNs) take center stage. RNNs emerge as a promising deep learning method for modeling time-sequential data by introducing recurrent connections between hidden units, establishing a link between historical patterns and current conditions. However, basic RNNs encounter challenges, particularly vanishing gradients, restricting their ability to process long-term information, known as the Long-Term Dependency problem. To address this, the Long Short-Term Memory (LSTM) technique is introduced. Illustrated in Figure 4.10 is a sample deep neural network featuring 50 LSTM units, showcasing the application of this solution to overcome the Long-Term Dependency problem.

Each LSTM block contains a cell state and three gates: namely input, forget, and the output gate. The input gate $i_t I_t$ is determined as

$$I_t = \beta\left(W_{PI}P_t + W_{HI}H_{t-1} + b_I\right)$$

where W is weight matrix, b bias vectors, and β logistic sigmoid function. The forget gate $f_t F$ can be expressed as

$$F_t = \beta\left(W_{PF}P_t + W_{HF}H_{t-1} + b_F\right).$$

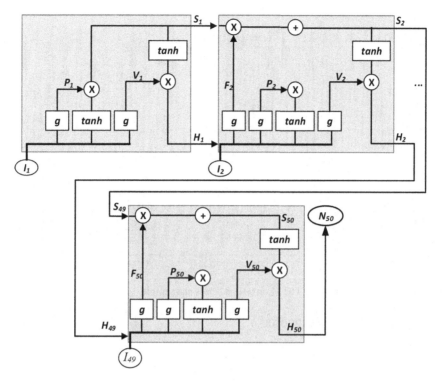

FIGURE 4.10   Basic architecture of a sample LSTM network.

The long-term memory is stored in a cell state vector S as expressed

$$S_t = F_t S_{t-1} + I_t \tanh\left(W_{PS}P_t + W_{HS}H_{t-1} + b_S\right).$$

The output gate O determines what is going to be an output as expressed as

$$V_t = \beta\left(W_{PV}P_t + W_{HV}H_{t-1} + b_V\right).$$

The hidden state H is expressed as

$$H_t = V_t \tanh\left(S_t\right).$$

Finally, the output U can be determined as

$$U = \text{softmax}\left(W_U H_l + b_U\right)$$

where l indicated the last LSTM number.

An example code of using LSTM for training and prediction of time-series data can be represented as follows and Figure 4.11 shows how efficient of LSTM can be to train and predict data.

```
import numpy as np
X_train = np.arange(0,100,0.5)
y_train = np.sin(X_train)
```

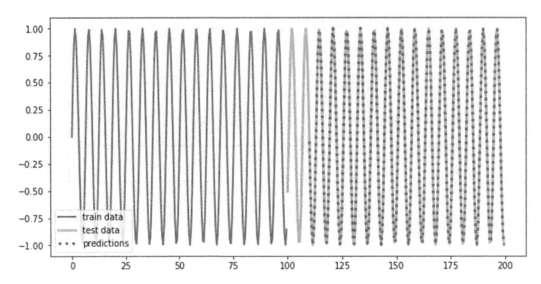

FIGURE 4.11   Result from applying LSTM on a time series test sample.

```
X _ test = np.arange(100,200,0.5)
y_test = np.sin(X_test)

n _ features = 1

train _ series = y _ train.reshape((len(y _ train), n _ features))
test_series = y_test.reshape((len(y_test), n_features))


from tensorflow.keras.preprocessing.sequence import
TimeseriesGenerator

train _ generator = TimeseriesGenerator(train _ series, train _ series,
                    length      = 20,
                    sampling_rate = 1,
                    stride      = 1,
                    batch_size  = 10)

test _ generator = TimeseriesGenerator(test _ series, test _ series,
                    length      = 20,
                    sampling_rate = 1,
                    stride      = 1,
                    batch_size  = 10)

from tensorflow.keras.models import Sequential
from tensorflow.keras.layers import Dense
from tensorflow.keras.layers import LSTM

model = Sequential()
model.add(LSTM(10, input_shape=(look_back, n_features)))
model.add(Dense(1))
model.compile(optimizer='adam', loss='mse')
```

```
model.fit(train _ generator,epochs=100, verbose=0)

test _ predictions = model.predict(test _ generator)

import matplotlib.pyplot as plt
x = np.arange(110,200,0.5)
fig, ax = plt.subplots(1, 1, figsize=(10, 5))
ax.plot(X_train,y_train, lw=2, label='train data')
ax.plot(X_test,y_test, lw=3, c='y', label='test data')
ax.plot(x,test_predictions, lw=3, c='g',linestyle = ':',
label='predictions')
ax.legend(loc="lower left")
plt.show();
```

4.3.4 Neural Structured Learning

Among the collection of deep learning tools, Google's open-source TensorFlow stands out as a widely utilized resource for modeling various events, particularly for prediction tasks related to pattern recognition. Complementing this, Neural Structured Learning (NSL) offers an open-source framework and represents one of the latest advancements in deep learning algorithms for understanding data events. NSL finds application in diverse research fields, including computer vision and natural language processing, where it proves valuable for constructing robust models. Functioning as a neural graph learning approach, NSL trains neural networks based on graphs and structured data. This method, emphasizing structured signals for training, generalizes adversarial learning by leveraging structured data with rich relational information among samples. It updates learning parameters using structured signals to ensure accurate learning while preserving input structure. Notably, NSL demonstrates superior performance in activity modeling and testing for activity recognition compared to traditional deep learning approaches like deep neural networks, CNNs, and RNNs. The neural structured learning approach, NSL, operates by incorporating structured signals alongside input features to effectively train neural networks. The algorithm prioritizes minimizing neighbors to uphold structural similarity in inputs, as reflected in the generalized neighbor loss equation provided.

$$\text{neigh}_{\text{loss}} = \sum_{k=0}^{W} L(y_{i,}\hat{y}_i) + \propto \sum_{k=0}^{W} L(y_{i,}x_{i,}N(x_i)).$$

The equation above leads to the conclusion that NSL extends the network in two distinct manners. In the initial scenario, neural graph learning is employed with neighbors represented through graphs. Conversely, in the second scenario, adversarial learning comes into play when neighbors are induced through adversarial perturbation.

As illustrated in Figure 4.12, the overall workflow of an NSL model for human activities is presented. Black arrows indicate the training process, while red arrows indicate the workflow in NSL using structured signals to optimize the model.

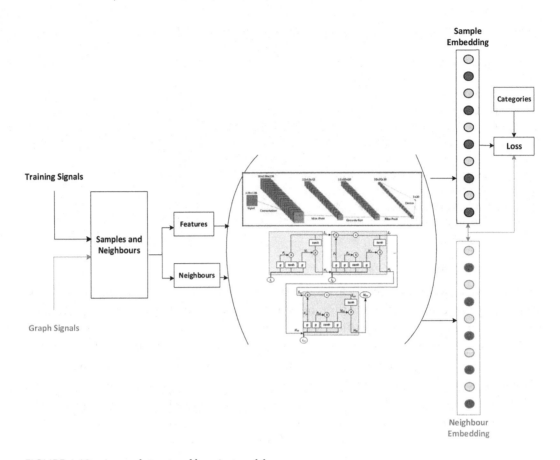

FIGURE 4.12   A neural structured learning model.

```
import tensorflow as tf
import neural_structured_learning as nsl

# Prepare data.
(x_train, y_train), (x_test, y_test) = tf.keras.datasets.mnist.
load_data()
x_train, x_test = x_train / 255.0, x_test / 255.0

# Create a base model -- sequential, functional, or subclass.
model = tf.keras.Sequential([
  tf.keras.Input((28, 28), name='feature'),
  tf.keras.layers.Flatten(),
  tf.keras.layers.Dense(128, activation=tf.nn.relu),
  tf.keras.layers.Dense(10, activation=tf.nn.softmax)
])

# Wrap the model with adversarial regularization.
adv_config = nsl.configs.make_adv_reg_config(multiplier=0.2,
adv_step_size=0.05)
adv_model = nsl.keras.AdversarialRegularization(model,
adv_config=adv_config)
```

```
# Compile, train, and evaluate.
adv_model.compile(optimizer='adam',
        loss='sparse_categorical_crossentropy',
        metrics=['accuracy'])
adv_model.fit({'feature': x_train, 'label': y_train}, batch_
size=32, epochs=5)
adv_model.evaluate({'feature': x_test, 'label': y_test})
```

The output represents 97% accuracy.

4.4 EXPLAINABLE AI (XAI)

Remarkable progress has been made by AI in the last decade, and, if managed and explored properly, it holds great potential for various applications [112–152. The artificial intelligence community is currently grappling with the challenge of explainability (XAI), which has become evident in the recent success of AI. XAI is crucial for practical applications of current AI models, prompting a need to deeply examine its contributions and focus on future prospects. AI researchers should prioritize trustworthy AI by exploring XAI for large-scale implementations, emphasizing explainability, fairness, and accountability. The success of machine learning models is largely attributed to efficient deep learning algorithms within vast parametric spaces, resulting in complex black-box models. The increased use of black-box machine learning models in critical contexts intensifies the demand for transparency, posing a risk of unjustifiable and illegitimate AI decisions. Therefore, explanations of a model's output become essential, especially in fields like precision medicine, assisted living, autonomous vehicles, finance, weather, medical emergencies, public safety, and security.

As demands for ethical AI increase, human acceptance becomes contingent on interpretable and trustworthy methods. Balancing performance and transparency of AI models is crucial, and improvements in interpretability and explainability can address model deficiencies. XAI aims to employ machine learning techniques to create more explainable models without compromising accuracy. Trustworthiness is considered a primary focus of XAI models, contributing to humans' understanding, trust, and effective management of AI phenomena. While all explainable models possess trustworthiness, not all trustworthy models are inherently explainable. The concept of trustworthiness is challenging to measure but plays a vital role in XAI research.

Explainability, as a social concept, ensures fairness in machine learning models. XAI models should illustrate how intermediary parameters affect output, addressing bias and emphasizing the fair or ethical analysis of these models. XAI can contribute to avoiding unethical usage of AI models as their applications expand, especially in sectors involving human lives. Privacy considerations are crucial for successful XAI models, as complex model structures and internal data representations may pose privacy risks. Ensuring the privacy and confidentiality of user data is paramount, particularly in critical sectors. Some researchers emphasize developing machine learning models that interact with users, a key factor in domains where user-centric decisions are predominant.

4.4.1 Local Explanations

Local explanations in AI models tackle explainability by partitioning the intricate solution space into simpler subspaces relevant to the entire model. Various methods with differentiating properties can be employed for basic model explanations, often representing limited sections of a model, falling into the category of local explanations. Rule extraction techniques, a majority based on model simplification, are commonly used. Local Interpretable Model-Agnostic Explanations (LIME) is a widely used method for local post-hoc explanation, generating local linear models to explain predictions of a complex machine learning model. LIME belongs to the category of rule-based local explanations through simplification. It constructs a new system based on the model to be explained and then designs a simplified model, aiming to maintain similar performance with reduced complexity. Figure 4.13 illustrates LIME's explanation of a test sample using a trained model, and Figure 4.14 showcases time-series prediction and explanation with LSTM model and LIME. Additionally, Figure 4.15 depicts LIME for visual explanations. The figures were generated using following XAI code of LIME.

```
import sklearn
import sklearn.datasets
import sklearn.ensemble
import numpy as np
import lime
import lime.lime_tabular

iris = sklearn.datasets.load _ iris()
train, test, labels_train, labels_test = sklearn.model_selection.
train_test_split(iris.data, iris.target, train_size=0.80)
rf = sklearn.ensemble.RandomForestClassifier(n_estimators=500)
rf.fit(train, labels_train)
sklearn.metrics.accuracy_score(labels_test, rf.predict(test))
```

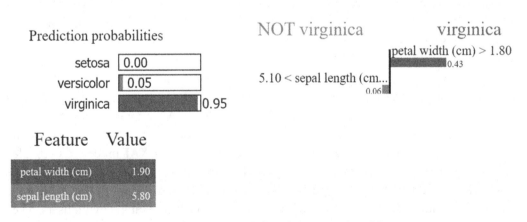

FIGURE 4.13   LIME example to explain a test sample based on a trained model.

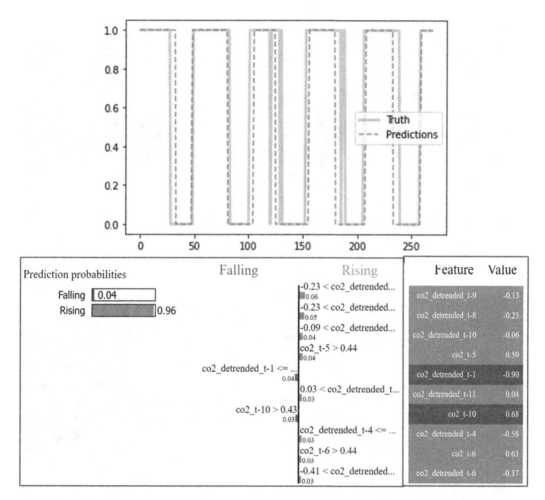

FIGURE 4.14 (top) Prediction of a time-series and (bottom) LIME explanation of a test sample based on a trained LSTM model.

```
explainer = lime.lime _ tabular.LimeTabularExplainer(train, feature _
names=iris.feature _ names, class _ names=iris.target _ names,
discretize _ continuous=True)
i = np.random.randint(0, test.shape[0])
exp = explainer.explain_instance(test[i], rf.predict_proba, num_
features=2, top_labels=1)

exp.show _ in _ notebook(show _ table=True, show _ all=False)

# Imports
import matplotlib.pyplot as plt
import numpy as np
import pandas as pd

from tensorflow.keras.models import Sequential
from tensorflow.keras.layers import LSTM, Dropout, Dense
```

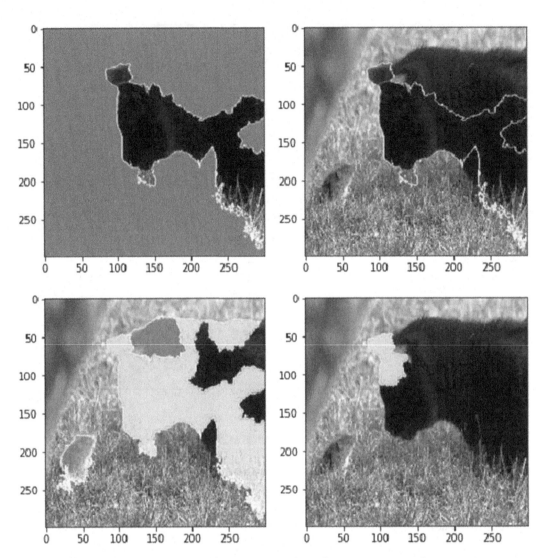

Figure 4.15   LIME explanation of a test image based on a pre-trained inception version 3.0 model.

```
from tensorflow.keras.optimizers import Adam
from tensorflow.keras.utils import to_categorical

from sklearn.preprocessing import MinMaxScaler
from sklearn.metrics import classification_report

from lime import lime_tabular

get_ipython().run_line_magic('matplotlib', 'inline')

#https://github.com/marcotcr/lime/blob/master/doc/notebooks/data/co2_
data.csv
```

```python
df = pd.read_csv('./co2_data.csv', index_col=0, parse_dates=True)

fig, (left, right) = plt.subplots(nrows=1, ncols=2, figsize=(13, 5))
df[['co2']].plot(ax=left)
df[['co2_detrended']].plot(ax=right)

def reshape_data(seq, n_timesteps):
  N = len(seq) - n_timesteps - 1
  nf = seq.shape[1]
  if N <= 0:
    raise ValueError('I need more data!')
  new_seq = np.zeros((N, n_timesteps, nf))
  for i in range(N):
    new_seq[i, :, :] = seq[i:i+n_timesteps]
  return new_seq

N_TIMESTEPS = 12 # Use 1 year of lookback

data_columns = ['co2', 'co2_detrended']
target_columns = ['rising']

from sklearn.preprocessing import MinMaxScaler
from tensorflow.keras.utils import to_categorical

scaler = MinMaxScaler(feature_range=(-1, 1))
X_original = scaler.fit_transform(df[data_columns].values)
X = reshape_data(X_original, n_timesteps=N_TIMESTEPS)
y = to_categorical((df[target_columns].values[N_TIMESTEPS:-1]).
astype(int))

# Train on the first 2000, and test on the last 276 samples
X_train = X[:2000]
y_train = y[:2000]
X_test = X[2000:]
y_test = y[2000:]
print(X.shape, y.shape)

model = Sequential()
model.add(LSTM(32, input_shape=(N_TIMESTEPS, len(data_columns))))
model.add(Dropout(0.2))
model.add(Dense(2, activation='softmax'))

optimizer = Adam(lr=1e-4)
model.compile(loss='binary_crossentropy', optimizer=optimizer)

model.fit(X_train, y_train, batch_size=100, epochs=500,
    validation_data=(X_test, y_test),
    verbose=1)

y_pred = np.argmax(model.predict(X_test), axis=1)
y_true = np.argmax(y_test, axis=1)
```

```
plt.plot(y_true, lw=3, alpha=0.3, label='Truth')
plt.plot(y_pred, '--', label='Predictions')
plt.legend(loc='best')

explainer = lime_tabular.RecurrentTabularExplainer(X_train,
training_labels=y_train, feature_names=data_columns,
                        discretize_continuous=True,
                        class_names=['Falling', 'Rising'],
                        discretizer='decile')

exp = explainer.explain_instance(X_test[50], model.predict, num_
features=10, labels=(1,))
exp.show_in_notebook()


import os
import keras
from tensorflow.keras.applications import inception_v3 as
inc_net
from tensorflow.keras.preprocessing import image
from tensorflow.keras.applications.imagenet_utils import
decode_predictions
from skimage.io import imread
import matplotlib.pyplot as plt
get_ipython().run_line_magic('matplotlib', 'inline')
import numpy as np

inet_model = inc_net.InceptionV3()

def transform_img_fn(path_list):
  out = []
  for img_path in path_list:
    img = image.load_img(img_path, target_size=(299, 299))
    x = image.img_to_array(img)
    x = np.expand_dims(x, axis=0)
    x = inc_net.preprocess_input(x)
    out.append(x)
  return np.vstack(out)

images = transform_img_fn([os.path.join('data','cat_mouse.jpg')])
# I'm dividing by 2 and adding 0.5 because of how this Inception
represents images
plt.imshow(images[0] / 2 + 0.5)
preds = inet_model.predict(images)
for x in decode_predictions(preds)[0]:
  print(x)

from lime import lime_image
```

```
explainer = lime _ image.LimeImageExplainer()

explanation = explainer.explain _ instance(images[0], inet _ model.
predict, top _ labels=5, hide _ color=0, num _ samples=1000)\n')

from skimage.segmentation import mark _ boundaries

temp, mask = explanation.get _ image _ and _ mask(explanation.top _
labels[0], positive _ only=True, num _ features=5, hide _ rest=False)
plt.imshow(mark_boundaries(temp / 2 + 0.5, mask))

temp, mask = explanation.get _ image _ and _ mask(explanation.top _
labels[0], positive _ only=False, num _ features=10, hide _ rest=False)
plt.imshow(mark_boundaries(temp / 2 + 0.5, mask))

temp, mask = explanation.get _ image _ and _ mask(explanation.
top _ labels[0], positive _ only=False, num _ features=1000, hide _
rest=False, min _ weight=0.1)

plt.imshow(mark _ boundaries(temp / 2 + 0.5, mask))
```

4.4.2 Visual Explanations

To address the explainability challenge in a model, textual explanations are crafted to elucidate the model's outcomes. These text explanations, along with visual explanations, aim to showcase the model's behavior using symbols that represent various strategies. Text explanations integrate each strategy into symbols that depict the model's functionality. Visualization techniques, coupled with dimensionality reduction methods, help obtain straightforward, human-interpretable visual representations. Alongside visualizations, other methods enhance comprehension, making them ideal for visually explaining complex models to users without an in-depth understanding of machine learning models. A visual explanation is crucial for acquiring model-agnostic explanations for artificial intelligence models. Recent research efforts have presented a portfolio of techniques, including global sensitivity analysis, to explain black-box models. Three novel sensitivity analysis methods—data-based, Monte-Carlo, and cluster-based—have been introduced, along with a novel measure of input importance, the average absolute deviation. Individual Conditional Expectation (ICE) plots are proposed for visualizing supervised machine learning models. In the field of model-agnostic methods for explaining post-hoc models, visual explanations are not as prevalent. Designing visualizations solely from inputs and outputs of an opaque machine learning model can be challenging, requiring seamless integration with any ML model, regardless of its internal structure. Therefore, visualization methods often combine with techniques assessing feature relevance to provide information for user display. The sample code below demonstrates using GradCAM for visual explanation, and Figures 4.16–4.22 showcases various outputs representing different explanations using following same Python code.

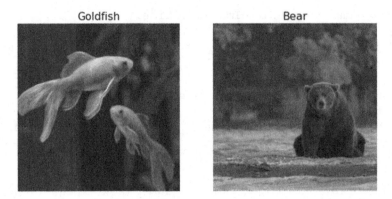

FIGURE 4.16   Two sample images to apply visual explanations based on VGG16 model.

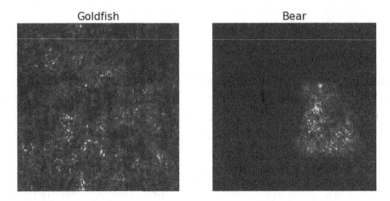

FIGURE 4.17   Vanilla saliency images applied on Figure 4.16.

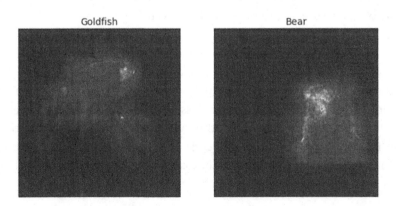

FIGURE 4.18   Smoothgrad saliency images applied on Figure 4.16.

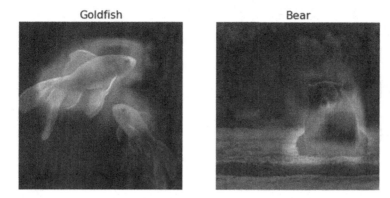

FIGURE 4.19   Generated heatmaps using GradCAM on Figure 4.16.

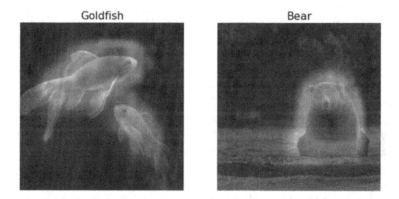

FIGURE 4.20   Generated heatmaps using GradCAM++ on Figure 4.16.

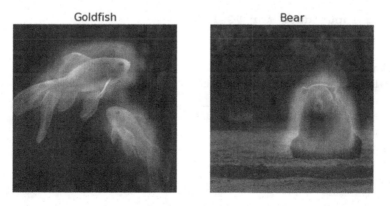

FIGURE 4.21   Generated heatmaps using ScoreCAM on Figure 4.16.

Goldfish

Bear

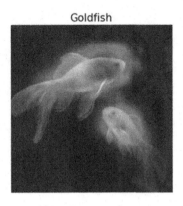 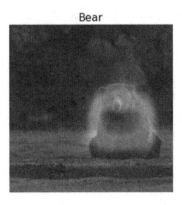

FIGURE 4.22   Generated heatmaps using Faster-ScoreCAM on Figure 4.16.

```python
import numpy as np
from matplotlib import pyplot as plt
import tensorflow as tf

from tensorflow.keras.applications.vgg16 import VGG16 as Model

model = Model(weights='imagenet', include_ top=True)

from tensorflow.keras.preprocessing.image import load_ img
from tensorflow.keras.applications.vgg16 import preprocess_input
image_titles = ['Goldfish', 'Bear']

# Load images and Convert them to a Numpy array
#https://github.com/keisen/tf-keras-vis/blob/master/docs/examples/
images/bear.jpg
#https://github.com/keisen/tf-keras-vis/blob/master/docs/examples/
images/goldfish.jpg

img1 = load_ img('./goldfish.jpg', target_ size=(224, 224))
img2 = load_img('./bear.jpg', target_size=(224, 224))
images = np.asarray([np.array(img1), np.array(img2)])

# Preparing input data for VGG16
X = preprocess_input(images)

# Rendering
f, ax = plt.subplots(nrows=1, ncols=2, figsize=(12, 4))
for i, title in enumerate(image_titles):
  ax[i].set_title(title, fontsize=16)
  ax[i].imshow(images[i])
  ax[i].axis('off')
plt.tight_layout()
plt.show()

from tf_ keras_ vis.utils.model_ modifiers import ReplaceToLinear
```

```
replace2linear = ReplaceToLinear()

# Instead of using the ReplaceToLinear instance above,
# you can also define the function from scratch as follows:
def model_modifier_function(cloned_model):
  cloned_model.layers[-1].activation = tf.keras.activations.linear

from tf_keras_vis.utils.scores import CategoricalScore

# 1 is the imagenet index corresponding to Goldfish, 294 to Bear.
score = CategoricalScore([1, 294])

# Instead of using CategoricalScore object,
# you can also define the function from scratch as follows:
def score_function(output):
  # The 'output' variable refers to the output of the model,
  # so, in this case, 'output' shape is '(3, 1000)' i.e.,
(samples, classes).
  return (output[0, 1], output[1, 294])

## Vanilla Saliency
%%time
from tensorflow.keras import backend as K
from tf_keras_vis.saliency import Saliency
# from tf_keras_vis.utils import normalize

# Create Saliency object.
saliency = Saliency(model,
          model_modifier=replace2linear,
          clone=True)

# Generate saliency map
saliency_map = saliency(score, X)

# saliency_map = normalize(saliency_map)

# Render
f, ax = plt.subplots(nrows=1, ncols=2, figsize=(12, 4))
for i, title in enumerate(image_titles):
  ax[i].set_title(title, fontsize=16)
  ax[i].imshow(saliency_map[i], cmap='jet')
  ax[i].axis('off')
plt.tight_layout()
plt.show()

## SmoothGrad
# Generate saliency map with smoothing that reduce noise by adding
noise
saliency_map = saliency(score,
          X,
```

```
            smooth_samples=20, # The number of calculating
gradients iterations.
            smooth_noise=0.20) # noise spread level.
```

```
# saliency_map = normalize(saliency_map)
```

```
# Render
f, ax = plt.subplots(nrows=1, ncols=2, figsize=(12, 4))
for i, title in enumerate(image_titles):
  ax[i].set_title(title, fontsize=14)
  ax[i].imshow(saliency_map[i], cmap='jet')
  ax[i].axis('off')
plt.tight_layout()
plt.show()
```

```
## GradCAM
from matplotlib import cm
from tf_keras_vis.gradcam import Gradcam
```

```
# Create Gradcam object
gradcam = Gradcam(model,
        model_modifier=replace2linear,
        clone=True)
```

```
# Generate heatmap with GradCAM
cam = gradcam(score,
      X,
      penultimate_layer=-1)
# Render
f, ax = plt.subplots(nrows=1, ncols=2, figsize=(12, 4))
for i, title in enumerate(image_titles):
  heatmap = np.uint8(cm.jet(cam[i])[…, :3] * 255)
  ax[i].set_title(title, fontsize=16)
  ax[i].imshow(images[i])
  ax[i].imshow(heatmap, cmap='jet', alpha=0.5) # overlay
  ax[i].axis('off')
plt.tight_layout()
plt.show()
```

```
## GradCAM++
```

```
from tf_keras_vis.gradcam_plus_plus import GradcamPlusPlus
# Create GradCAM++ object
gradcam = GradcamPlusPlus(model,
            model_modifier=replace2linear,
            clone=True)
# Generate heatmap with GradCAM++
cam = gradcam(score,
      X,
      penultimate_layer=-1)
```

```
f, ax = plt.subplots(nrows=1, ncols=2, figsize=(12, 4))
for i, title in enumerate(image_titles):
  heatmap = np.uint8(cm.jet(cam[i])[…, :3] * 255)
  ax[i].set_title(title, fontsize=16)
  ax[i].imshow(images[i])
  ax[i].imshow(heatmap, cmap='jet', alpha=0.5)
  ax[i].axis('off')
plt.tight_layout()
plt.savefig('./gradcam_plus_plus.png')
plt.show()


## ScoreCAM
from tf_keras_vis.scorecam import Scorecam
from tf_keras_vis.utils import num_of_gpus


# Create ScoreCAM object
scorecam = Scorecam(model)


# Generate heatmap with ScoreCAM
cam = scorecam(score, X, penultimate_layer=-1)


## Since v0.6.0, calling `normalize()` is NOT necessary.
# cam = normalize(cam)


# Render
f, ax = plt.subplots(nrows=1, ncols=2, figsize=(12, 4))
for i, title in enumerate(image_titles):
  heatmap = np.uint8(cm.jet(cam[i])[…, :3] * 255)
  ax[i].set_title(title, fontsize=16)
  ax[i].imshow(images[i])
  ax[i].imshow(heatmap, cmap='jet', alpha=0.5)
  ax[i].axis('off')
plt.tight_layout()
plt.show()


## Faster-ScoreCAM

from tf _ keras _ vis.scorecam import Scorecam


# Create ScoreCAM object
scorecam = Scorecam(model, model_modifier=replace2linear)


# Generate heatmap with Faster-ScoreCAM
cam = scorecam(score,
        X,
        penultimate_layer=-1,
        max_N=10)


## Since v0.6.0, calling `normalize()` is NOT necessary.
# cam = normalize(cam)
```

```
# Render
f, ax = plt.subplots(nrows=1, ncols=2, figsize=(12, 4))
for i, title in enumerate(image_titles):
  heatmap = np.uint8(cm.jet(cam[i])[..., :3] * 255)
  ax[i].set_title(title, fontsize=16)
  ax[i].imshow(images[i])
  ax[i].imshow(heatmap, cmap='jet', alpha=0.5)
  ax[i].axis('off')
plt.tight_layout()
plt.show()
```

4.4.3 Feature Relevance Explanations

Feature relevance explanation techniques for explainability unveil the internal structural workings of a model by computing relevance scores for the variable parameters. These scores measure the sensitivity of a feature to the model's output, illustrating the significant role variables play in the modeling process. Typically employed to elucidate the functioning of an opaque model, feature relevance explanation methods rank the influence, relevance, and importance of specific features on model predictions. A notable contribution to this domain is SHapley Additive exPlanations (SHAP), offering a method to calculate feature importance scores for individual predictions with desirable properties such as local accuracy, missingness, and consistency. Leveraging coalitional game theory and local gradients, researchers achieved properties absent in previous methods. Local gradients also test changes in the model's output. In alignment with research in other domains, feature relevance techniques have become a pivotal exploration area in the current landscape of explainable artificial intelligence. Following code is to apply SHAP on ResNet50 following explanations in Figure 4.23.

```
import json
from tensorflow.keras.applications.resnet50 import ResNet50,
preprocess_input
import shap

# load pre-trained model and choose two images to explain
model = ResNet50(weights="imagenet")

def f(X):
  tmp = X.copy()
  preprocess_input(tmp)
  return model(tmp)

X, y = shap.datasets.imagenet50()

# load the ImageNet class names as a vectorized mapping function
from ids to names
url = "https://s3.amazonaws.com/deep-learning-models/image-models/
imagenet_class_index.json"
with open(shap.datasets.cache(url)) as file:
  class_names = [v[1] for v in json.load(file).values()]
```

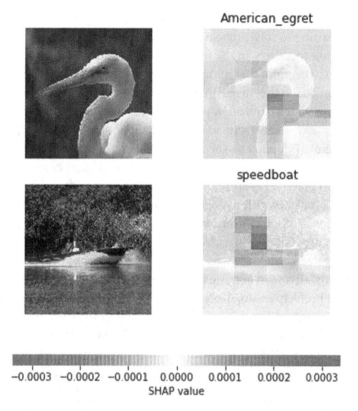

FIGURE 4.23   Two sample image classification and SHAP explanations after using Resnet50 pre-trained model on them.

```
# define a masker that is used to mask out partitions of the input
image, this one uses a blurred background
masker = shap.maskers.Image("inpaint _ telea", X[0].shape)

# By default the Partition explainer is used for all partition
explainer
explainer = shap.Explainer(f, masker, output_names=class_names)

# here we use 500 evaluations of the underlying model to estimate
the SHAP values
shap_values = explainer(
  X[1:3], max_evals=500, batch_size=50, outputs=shap.Explanation.
argsort.flip[:1]
)
shap.image_plot(shap_values)
```

4.5 CONCLUSION

As many sectors embrace new information technologies these days, machine learning is at the center of these technologies. In spite of the fact that the origins of machine learning can be traced back many decades, a clear consensus has emerged regarding the supreme significance of intelligent machines equipped with the ability to learn, reason, and adapt. There is no doubt that machine learning methods have been achieving unprecedented levels of performance when learning to solve increasingly complex computational tasks, making them of critical importance to society in the future. Machine learning-powered architecture has recently advanced to the point that many practical applications can be performed without human intervention due to the increasing sophistication of these architectures. The goal of this chapter was to provide an overview of different machine learning techniques consisting of shallow and deep architectures, in addition to a discussion of pre-trained huge machine learning models, mostly applied to successful image recognition applications. The entire chapter has demonstrated that shallow machine learning techniques are mostly transparent and easy to apply in practical applications; however, they are not as efficient when applied to highly complex problems with massive amounts of data, where deep learning provides significant advantages. Although deep learning techniques have gained significant momentum and have been appropriately harnessed, they may be able to deliver the best results in many sectors and research fields when appropriately applied. In order for this to occur in deep learning shortly, all researchers must overcome the barrier of transparency and explain ability, an inherent problem arising from the latest techniques used in deep learning. It has been noted that the solutions to this problem are found in the eXplainable AI (XAI) field, which is recognized as an important element for the deployment of ML models in practical and vital applications. Therefore, several XAI techniques have been explored. Thus, this chapter has discussed different machine learning algorithms including shallow and deep ones. In addition, it also has tried to explain different XAI techniques with examples.

REFERENCES

[1] H. Moosaei, S. Ketabchi, M. Razzaghi, and M. Tanveer, "Generalized Twin Support Vector Machines," *Neural Processing Letters*, vol. 53, pp. 1545–1564, 2021.

[2] O. L. Mangasarian, "Data Mining via Support Vector Machines," in: *Proceedings of the IFIP Conference on System Modeling and Optimization*, Trier, Germany, July 23–27 2001, pp. 91–112.

[3] Y. J. Lee and O. L. Mangasarian, "SSVM: A Smooth Support Vector Machine for Classification," *Computational Optimization and Applications*, vol. 20, pp. 5–22, 2001.

[4] M. Choi, G. Koo, M. Seo, and S. W. Kim, "Wearable Device-Based System to Monitor a Driver's Stress, Fatigue, and Drowsiness," *IEEE Transactions on Instrumentation and Measurement*, vol. 67, pp. 634–645, 2018.

[5] S. Ortega, H. Fabelo, M. Halicek, R. Camacho, M. D. L. L. Plaza, G. M. Callicó, and B. Fei, "Hyperspectral Superpixel-wise Glioblastoma Tumor Detection in Histological Samples," *Applied Sciences*, vol. 10, pp. 4448, 2020.

[6] S. Setiowati, E. L. Franita, and I. Ardiyanto, "A Review of Optimization Method in Face Recognition: Comparison Deep Learning and Non-deep Learning Methods," in: *Proceedings of the 9th International Conference on Information Technology and Electrical Engineering (ICITEE)*, Phuket, Thailand, October 12–13 2017, pp. 1–6.

[7] R. Pandit and A. Kolios, "SCADA Data-Based Support Vector Machine Wind Turbine Power Curve Uncertainty Estimation and Its Comparative Studies," *Applied Science*, vol. 10, p. 8685, 2020.

[8] A. Rizwan, N. Iqbal, R. Ahmad, and D. H. Kim, "WR-SVM Model Based on the Margin Radius Approach for Solving the Minimum Enclosing Ball Problem in Support Vector Machine Classification," *Applied Science*, vol. 11, p. 4657, 2021.

[9] R. Muzzammel and A. Raza, "A Support Vector Machine Learning-Based Protection Technique for MT-HVDC Systems," *Energies*, vol. 13, p. 6668, 2020, doi: https://doi.org/10.3390/en132 46668

[10] D. Van Hertem, O. Gomis-Bellmunt, and J. Liang, *HVDC Grids: For Offshore and Supergrid of the Future*; John Wiley & Sons: Hoboken, NJ, USA, 2016, pp. 1–528.

[11] M. Callavik, A. Blomberg, J. Häfner, and B. Jacobson, "Break-Through!: ABB's Hybrid HVDC Breaker, an Innovation Breakthrough Enabling Reliable HVDC Grids," *ABB Grid Systems*, 2013.

[12] V.N. Vapnik, *Statistical Learning Theory*; Wiley: New York, NY, USA, 1998, p. 736.

[13] C. Cortes and V. Vapnik, "Support-Vector Networks," *Machine Learning*, vol. 20, pp. 273–297, 1995.

[14] S. Haykin, *Neural Networks: A Comprehensive Foundation*, 2nd ed.; Prentice Hall PTR: Upper Saddle River, NJ, USA, 1998, p. 842.

[15] J. Ren, "ANN vs. SVM: Which One Performs Better in Classification of MCCs in Mammogram Imaging," *Knowledge-based Systems*, vol. 26, 144–153, 2012.

[16] X. Wu, D. Wang, W. Cao, and M. Ding, "A Genetic-Algorithm Support Vector Machine and D-S Evidence Theory Based Fault Diagnostic Model for Transmission Line," *IEEE Transactions on Power Systems*, vol. 34, pp. 4186–4194, 2019.

[17] M. Zhang and H. Wang, "Fault Location for MMC–MTDC Transmission Lines Based on Least Squares-Support Vector Regression," *Journal of Engineering*, vol. 2019, pp. 2125–2130, 2019.

[18] H. Lala, S. Karmakar, and A.K. Singh, "MATLAB-Based GUI Development for the Detection and Localization of Faults in Transmission Line," in: *Proceedings of the IEEE Region 10 Symposium (TENSYMP)*, Kolkata, India, 20–22 December 2019; IEEE: Kolkata, India; pp. 654–659.

[19] Q. Wang, Y. Yu, H.O.A. Ahmed, M. Darwish, and A.K. Nandi, "Fault Detection and Classification in MMC-HVDC Systems Using Learning Methods," *Sensors*, vol. 20, p. 4438, 2020.

[20] H.R. Baghaee, D. Mlakić, S. Nikolovski, and T. Dragicević, "Support Vector Machine-Based Islanding and Grid Fault Detection in Active Distribution Networks," *IEEE Journal of Emerging and Selected Topics in Power Electronics*, vol. 8, pp. 2385–2403, 2020.

[21] H. R. Baghaee, D. Mlakić, S. Nikolovski, and T. Dragičević, "Anti-islanding Protection of PV-Based Microgrids Consisting of PHEVs Using SVMs," *IEEE Transactions on Smart Grid*, vol. 11, pp. 483–500, 2020.

[22] M. Sheykhmousa, M. Mahdianpari, H. Ghanbari, F. Mohammadimanesh, P. Ghamisi, and S. Homayouni, "Support Vector Machine vs. Random Forest for Remote Sensing Image Classification: A Meta-Analysis and Systematic Review," *IEEE Journal of Selected Topics in Applied Earth Observations and Remote Sensing*, vol. 13, p. 18, 2020.

[23] T. M. Berhane, C. R. Lane, Q. Wu, B. C. Autrey, O. A. Anenkhonov, V. V. Chepinoga, and H. Liu, "Decision-Tree, Rule-Based, and Random Forest Classification of High-Resolution Multispectral Imagery for Wetland Mapping and Inventory," *Remote Sensing*, vol. 10, p. 580, 2018.

[24] J. Hatwell, M. M. Gaber, and R. M. A. Azad, "CHIRPS: Explaining Random Forest Classification," *Artificial Intelligence Review*, vol. 53, pp. 5747–5788, 2020.

[25] R. Genuer, J. -M. Poggi, and C. Tuleau-Malot, "Variable Selection Using Random Forests," *Pattern Recognition Letters*, vol. 31, no. 14, pp. 2225–2236, 2010.

[26] M. Haddouchi and A. Berrado, in: *A survey of methods and tools used for interpreting random forest 2019 1st International Conference on Smart Systems and Data Science (ICSSD)*, IEEE, 2019, pp. 1–6.

[27] X. Zhao, Y. Wu, D. L. Lee, and W. Cui, "Iforest: Interpreting Random Forests via Visual Analytics," *IEEE Transactions on Visualization and Computer Graphics*, vol. 25, no. 1, pp. 407–416, 2018.

[28] V. A. de Freitas Barbosa, J. C. Gomes, M. A. de Santana, C. L. de Lima, R. B. Calado, C. R. Bertoldo, Jr., J. E. de Almeida Albuqurque, R. G. de Souza, R. J. E. de Araujo, R. E. de Souza, et al., Covid-19 Rapid Test by Combining a Random Forest Based Web System and Blood Tests, medRxiv 2020.

[29] V. K. Gupta, D. Kumar, and A. Sardana, "Prediction of COVID-19 Confirmed, Death, and Cured Cases in India Using Random Forest Model," *Big Data Mining and Analytics*, vol. 4, pp. 116–123, 2021.

[30] C. M. Yesilkanat, "Spatio-temporal Estimation of the Daily Cases of COVID-19 in Worldwide Using Random Forest Machine Learning Algorithm," *Chaos Solitons Fractals*, vol. 140, p. 110210, 2020.

[31] C. An, H. Lim, D. W. Kim, J. H. Chang, Y. J. Choi, and S. W. Kim, "Machine Learning Prediction for Mortality of Patients Diagnosed with COVID-19: A Nationwide Korean Cohort Study," *Science Report*, vol. 10, p. 18716, 2020.

[32] J. Wang, H. Yu, Q. Hua, S. Jing, Z. Liu, X. Peng, C. Cao, and Y. Luo, "A Descriptive Study of Random Forest Algorithm for Predicting COVID-19 Patients Outcome," *PeerJ*, vol. 8, p. e9945, 2020.

[33] R. Majhi, R. Thangeda, R. P. Sugasi, and N. Kumar, "Analysis and Prediction of COVID-19 Trajectory: A Machine Learning Approach," *Journal of Public Affairs*, vol. 21, p. e2537, 2020.

[34] Z. Tang, W. Zhao, X. Xie, Z. Zhong, F. Shi, J. Liu, and D. Shen, Severity Assessment of Coronavirus Disease 2019 (COVID-19) Using Quantitative Features from Chest CT Images, 2020 arXiv, arXiv:2003.11988.

[35] V. A. de Freitas Barbosa, J. C. Gomes, M. A. de Santana, C. L. de Lima, R. B. Calado, C. R. Bertoldo, Jr., J. E. de Almeida Albuqurque, R. G. de Souza, R. J. E. de Araujo, R. E. de Souza, et al., COVID-19 Rapid Test by Combining a Random Forest Based Web System and Blood Tests, medRxiv, 2020.

[36] V. K. Gupta, D. Kumar, and A. Sardana, "Prediction of COVID-19 Confirmed, Death, and Cured Cases in India Using Random Forest Model," *Big Data Mining and Analytics*, vol. 4, p. 116–123, 2021.

[37] C. M. Yesilkanat, "Spatio-temporal Estimation of the Daily Cases of COVID-19 in Worldwide Using Random Forest Machine Learning Algorithm," *Chaos Solitons Fractals*, vol. 140, p. 110210, 2020.

[38] C. An, H. Lim, D. W. Kim, J. H. Chang, Y. J. Choi, and S. W. Kim, "Machine Learning Prediction for Mortality of Patients Diagnosed with COVID-19: A Nationwide Korean Cohort Study," *Science Report*, vol. 10, p. 18716, 2020.

[39] J. Wang, H. Yu, Q. Hua, S. Jing, Z. Liu, X. Peng, C. Cao, and Y. Luo, "A Descriptive Study of Random Forest Algorithm for Predicting COVID-19 Patients Outcome," *PeerJ*, vol. 8, p. e9945, 2020.

[40] R. Majhi, R. Thangeda, R. P. Sugasi, and N. Kumar, "Analysis and Prediction of COVID-19 Trajectory: A Machine Learning Approach," *Journal of Public Affairs*, vol. 21, p. e2537, 2020.

[41] C. Bentéjac, A. Csörgő, and G. Martínez-Muñoz, "A Comparative Analysis of Gradient Boosting Algorithms," *Artificial Intelligence Review*, vol. 54, pp. 1937–1967, 2021, https://doi.org/10.1007/s10462-020-09896-5

[42] E. Yaman and A. Subasi, "Comparison of Band Boosting Ensemble Machine Learning Methods for Automated EMG Signal Classification," *BioMed Research International*, vol. 2019, pp. 1–13, 2019.

[43] E. G. Dada, J. S. Bassi, H. Chiroma, A. O. Adetunmbi, and O. E. Ajibuwa, "Machine Learning for Email Spam Filtering: Review Approaches and Open Research Problems," *Heliyon*, vol. 5, no. 6, pp. e01802, 2019.

[44] D.-K. Thai, T. M. Tu, T. Q. Bui, and T.-T. Bui, "Gradient Tree Boosting Machine Learning on Predicting the Failure Modes of the RC Panels Under Impact Loads," *Engineering with Computers*, vol. 37, no. 1, pp. 1–12, 2019.

[45] S. Nawar and A. M. Mouazen, "Comparison Between Random Forests Artificial Neural Networks and Gradient Boosted Machines Methods of On-Line Vis-NIR Spectroscopy Measurements of Soil Total Nitrogen and Total Carbon," *Sensors*, vol. 17, no. 10, pp. 2428, 2017.

[46] K. S. Hoon, K. C. Yeo, S. Azam, B. Shunmugam, and F. De Boer, "Critical Review of Machine Learning Approaches to Apply Big Data Analytics in DDoS Forensics," in: *2018 International Conference on Computer Communication and Informatics (ICCCI)*, 2018, pp. 1–5.

[47] X. Tong, *Breast Cancer Prediction from Genome Segments with Machine Learning*, University of California, Irvine, 2018.

[48] D. Nielsen, *Tree Boosting with XGBoost—Why Does XGBoost win "Every" Machine Learning Competition?*, NTNU, 2016.

[49] Y. Xia, C. Liu, Y. Li, and N. Liu, "A Boosted Decision Tree Approach Using Bayesian Hyper-parameter Optimization for Credit Scoring," *Expert Systems with Applications*, vol. 78, pp. 225–241, 2017.

[50] E. Al Daoud, "Comparison between XGBoost LightGBM and CatBoost Using a Home Credit Dataset," *International Journal of Computer and Information Engineering*, vol. 13, no. 1, pp. 6–10, 2019.

[51] G. Ke, Q. Meng, T. Finley, T. Wang, W. Chen, W. Ma, Q. Ye, T. Y. Liu, "Lightgbm: A Highly Efficient Gradient Boosting Decision Tree," *Advances in Neural Information Processing Systems*, vol. 30, pp. 3146–3154, 2017.

[52] I. Babajide Mustapha and F. Saeed, , "Bioactive Molecule Prediction Using Extreme Gradient Boosting," *Molecules*, vol. 21, no. 8, p. 983, 2016.

[53] T. Chen and C. Guestrin, "Xgboost: A Scalable Tree Boosting System," in: *Proceedings of the 22nd ACM SIGKDD International Conference on Knowledge Discovery and Data Mining, KDD'16*; ACM: New York, NY, USA, pp. 785–794, 2016.

[54] T. G. Dieterich. "An Experimental Comparison of Three Methods for Constructing Ensembles of Decision Trees: Bagging, Boosting, and Randomization," *Machine Learning*, vol. 40, no. 2, pp. 139–157, 2000.

[55] J. H. Friedman, "Greedy Function Approximation: A Gradient Boosting Machine," *Annals of Statistics*, vol. 29, no. 5, pp. 1189–1232, 2001.

[56] J. H. Friedman, "Stochastic Gradient Boosting," *Computational Statistics and Data Analysis*, vol. 38, no. 4, pp. 367–378, 2002.

[57] M. Gumus and M. S. Kiran, "Crude Oil Price Forecasting Using XGBoost," in *2017 International Conference on Computer Science and Engineering (UBMK)*, pp. 1100–1103, 2002.

[58] G. Ke, Q. Meng, T. Finley, T. Wang, W. Chen, W. Ma, Q. Ye, and T. Y. Liu, "Lightgbm: A Highly Efficient Gradient Boosting Decision Tree," in: I. Guyon, U.V. Luxburg, S. Bengio, H. Wallach, R. Fergus, S. Vishwanathan, and R. Garnett, Eds, *Advances in Neural Information Processing Systems*, vol 30, pp 3146–3154, 2018.

[59] L. Prokhorenkova, G. Gusev, A. Vorobev, A. V. Dorogush, and A. Gulin, "Catboost: Unbiased Boosting with Categorical Features," in: S. Bengio, H. Wallach, H. Larochelle, K. Grauman, N. Cesa-Bianchi, and R. Garnett, Eds, *Advances in Neural Information Processing Systems*, vol 31, pp 6638–6648, 2018.

[60] Y. Xia, C. Liu, Y. Li, and N. Liu, "A Boosted Decision Tree Approach Using Bayesian Hyper-parameter Optimization for Credit Scoring. *Expert Systems with Applications*, vol. 78, pp. 225–241, 2017.

[61] R. E. S. Yoav Freund, "A Short Introduction to Boosting," *Japanese Society for Artificial Intelligence*, vol. 14, no. 5, pp. 771–780, 1999.

[62] J. Javid, M. A. Mughal, and M. Karim, "Using kNN Algorithm for Classification of Distribution Transformers Health Index," in: *2021 International Conference on Innovative Computing (ICIC)*, 2021, pp. 1–6, doi: 10.1109/ICIC53490.2021.9693013

[63] A. Moldagulova and R. B. Sulaiman, "Using KNN Algorithm for Classification of Textual Documents," in: *ICIT 2017 – 8th International Conference on Information Technology*, pp. 665–671, 2017.

[64] Y. Li and B. Cheng, "An Improved k-Nearest Neighbor Algorithm and Its Application to High Resolution Remote Sensing Image Classification," in: *2009 17th International Conference on Geoinformatics 2009*, 2009, pp. 1–4.

[65] S. Taneja, C. Gupta, K. Goyal, and D. Gureja, "An Enhanced K-Nearest Neighbor Algorithm Using Information Gain and Clustering," in: *International Conference on Advanced Computing and Communication Technology, ACCT*, 2014, pp. 325–329.

[66] F. Pedregosa, G. Varoquaux, A. Gramfort, V. Michel, B. Thirion, O. Grisel, M. Blondel, P. Prettenhofer, R. Weiss, V. Dubourg, J. Verplas, A. Passos, D. Cournapeau, M. Brucher, M. Perrot, and E. Duchesnay, "Scikit-Learn: Machine Learning in Python," *Journal of Machine Learning Research*, vol. 12, pp. 2825–2830, 2011.

[67] G. E. Hinton, "Deep Belief Networks," *Scholarpedia*, vol. 4, no. 5, pp. 5947, 2009.

[68] Y. Zeng, T. Dong, Q. Pei, J. Liu, and J. Ma, "LPDBN: A Privacy Preserving Scheme for Deep Belief Network," in: *IEEE INFOCOM 2021 – IEEE Conference on Computer Communications Workshops (INFOCOM WKSHPS)*, 2021, pp. 1–6, doi: 10.1109/INFOCOMWKSHPS51825.2021.9484592

[69] P. Zhang, X. Kang, D. Wu, and R. Wang, "High-Accuracy Entity State Prediction Method Based on Deep Belief Network Toward IoT Search," *IEEE Wireless Communications Letters*, vol. 8, no. 2, pp. 492–495, April 2019.

[70] Y. Qin, X. Wang, and J. Zou, "The Optimized Deep Belief Networks with Improved Logistic Sigmoid Units and Their Application in Fault Diagnosis for Planetary Gearboxes of Wind Turbines," *IEEE Transactions on Industrial Electronics*, vol. 66, no. 5, pp. 3814–3824, May 2019.

[71] T. Ouyang, Y. He, H. Li, Z. Sun, and S. Baek, "Modeling and Forecasting Short-Term Power Load with Copula Model and Deep Belief Network," *IEEE Transactions on Emerging Topics in Computational Intelligence*, vol. 3, no. 2, pp. 127–136, April 2019.

[72] C. Zhang, K. C. Tan, H. Li, and G. S. Hong, "A Cost-Sensitive Deep Belief Network for Imbalanced Classification," *IEEE Transactions on Neural Networks and Learning Systems*, vol. 30, no. 1, pp. 109–122, Jan. 2019.

[73] J. Konecny, H. B. McMahan, F.X. Yu, P. Richtárik, A.T. Suresh, and D. Bacon, Federated Learning: Strategies for Improving Communication Efficiency", 2016, arXiv preprint, arXiv: 1610.05492.

[74] H. Lee, R. Grosse, R. Ranganath, Y. N. Andrew, "Convolutional Deep Belief Networks for Scalable Unsupervised Learning of Hierarchical Representations", in: *Proceedings of the 26th Annual International Conference on Machine Learning*, 2009, pp. 609–616.

[75] N. H. Phan, X. Wu, and D. Dou, "Preserving Differential Privacy in Convolutional Deep Belief Networks," *Machine Learning*, vol. 106, no. 9–10, pp. 1681–1704, 2017.

[76] C. Gianoglio, E. Ragusa, R. Zunino, and M. Valle, "1-D Convolutional Neural Networks for Touch Modalities Classification," in: *2021 28th IEEE International Conference on Electronics, Circuits, and Systems (ICECS)*, 2021, pp. 1–6, doi: 10.1109/ICECS53924.2021.9665576

[77] Z. Lei, J. Xie, and L. Xiao, "Inertial Sensor-based Human Activity Recognition Using Hybrid Deep Neural Networks," in: *2021 14th International Congress on Image and Signal Processing, BioMedical Engineering and Informatics (CISP-BMEI)*, 2021, pp. 1–7, doi: 10.1109/ CISP-BMEI53629.2021.9624347

[78] A. Dhillon and G. K. Verma, "Convolutional Neural Network: A Review of Models Methodologies and Applications to Object Detection," *Progress in Artificial Intelligence*, vol. 9, pp. 85–112, 2020.

[79] J. Ker, L. Wang, J. Rao, and T. Lim, "Deep Learning Applications in Medical Image Analysis", *IEEE Access*, vol. 6, pp. 9375–9389, 2018.

[80] M. M. Badza and M. Barjaktarovi, "Classification of Brain Tumors from MRI Images Using a Convolutional Neural Network", *Applied Sciences*, vol. 10, no. 6, pp. 1999(1–13), 2020.

[81] S. S. Yadav and S. M. Jadhav, "Deep Convolutional Neural Network Based Medical Image Classification for Disease Diagnosis," *Journal of Big Data*, vol. 6, no. 1, pp. 113(1–18), 2019.

[82] J. Ker, S. P. Singh, Y. Bai, J. Rao, T. Lim, and L. Wang, "Image Thresholding Improves 3-Dimensional Convolutional Neural Network Diagnosis of Different Acute Brain Hemorrhages on Computed Tomography Scans", *Sensors*, vol. 19, no. 9, pp. 2167(1–12), 2019.

[83] S. P. Singh, L. Wang, S. Gupta, B. Gulyas, and P. Padmanabhan, "Shallow 3D CNN for Detecting Acute Brain Hemorrhage from Medical Imaging Sensors," *IEEE Sensors Journal*, vol. 21, no. 13, pp. 14290–14299, 2021.

[84] S. P. Singh, L. Wang, S. Gupta, and H. Goli, "3D Deep Learning on Medical Images: A Review," *Sensors*, vol. 20, no. 18, pp. 5097(1–24), 2020.

[85] W. A. Kusuma, A. E. Minarno, and M. S. Wibowo, "Triaxial Accelerometer-Based Human Activity Recognition Using 1D Convolution Neural Network," in: *2020 International Workshop on Big Data and Information Security (IWBIS)*, 2020, pp. 53–58.

[86] K. Wang, J. He, and L. Zhang, "Attention-Based Convolutional Neural Network for Weakly Labeled Human Activities' Recognition with Wearable Sensors," *IEEE Sensors Journal*, vol. 19, no. 17, pp. 7598–7604, 2019.

[87] B. Lindemann, T. Müller, H. Vietz, N. Jazdi, and M. Weyrich, "A Survey on Long Short-Term Memory Networks for Time Series Prediction," *Procedia CIRP*, vol. 99, pp. 650–655, 2021.

[88] J. L. Leevy and T. M. Khoshgoftaar, "A Short Survey of LSTM Models for De-identification of Medical Free Text," in: *2020 IEEE 6th International Conference on Collaboration and Internet Computing (CIC)*, 2020, pp. 117–124, doi: 10.1109/CIC50333.2020.00023

[89] X. Ma, J. Zhang, B. Du, C. Ding, and L. Sun, "Parallel Architecture of Convolutional Bi-Directional LSTM Neural Networks for Network-Wide Metro Ridership Prediction," *IEEE Transactions on Intelligent Transportation Systems*, vol. 20, no. 6, pp. 2278–2288, ,2018.

[90] H. Xue, Q. Du Huynh, and M. Reynolds, "SS-LSTM: A Hierarchical LSTM Model for Pedestrian Trajectory Prediction," in: *2018 IEEE Winter Conference on Applications of Computer Vision (WACV)*, 2018, pp. 1186–1194.

[91] K.-F. Chu, A. Y. S. Lam, V. O. K. Li, "Deep Multi-scale Convolutional LSTM Network for Travel Demand and Origin-Destination Predictions," *IEEE Transactions on Intelligent Transportation Systems*, vol. 21, no. 8, pp. 3219–3232, 2019.

[92] C.-J. Huang and P.-H. Kuo, "A Deep CNN-LSTM Model for Particulate Matter (PM2. 5) Forecasting in Smart Cities." *Sensors*, vol. 18, no. 7, pp. 1-22, 2018.

[93] T.-Y. Kim and S.-B. Cho, "Predicting Residential Energy Consumption Using CNN-LSTM Neural Networks," *Energy*, vol. 182, pp. 72–81, 2019.

[94] A. Gensler, J. Henze, B. Sick, and N. Raabe, "Deep Learning for Solar Power Forecasting—An Approach Using AutoEncoder and LSTM Neural Networks," in: *2016 IEEE international conference on systems, man, and cybernetics (SMC)*, pp. 2858–2865, 2016.

[95] B. Lindemann, N. Jazdi, and M. Weyrich, "Detektion von Anomalien zur Qualitätssicherung basierend auf Sequence-to-Sequence LSTM Netzen," *at-Automatisierungstechnik*, vol. 67, no. 12, pp. 1058–1068, 2019.

[96] S. Du, T. Li, and S.-J. Horng, "Time Series Forecasting Using Sequence-to-Sequence Deep Learning Framework," in: *2018 9th International Symposium on Parallel Architectures, Algorithms and Programming (PAAP)*, 2018, pp. 171–176.

[97] A. Gopalan, D. -C. Juan, C. I. Magalhaes, C. -S. Ferng, A. Heydon, C. -T. Lu, P. Pham, G. Yu, Y. Fan, and Y. Wang, "Neural Structured Learning: Training Neural Networks with Structured Signals," in: *Proceedings of the 14th ACM International Conference on Web Search and Data Mining (WSDM '21)*; Association for Computing Machinery: New York, NY, USA, 2021, pp. 1150–1153. https://doi.org/10.1145/3437963.3441666

[98] Neural Structured Learning in TensorFlow, 2019. https://www.tensorflow.org/neural_structured_learning

[99] M. Abadi, A. Agarwal, P. Barham, E. Brevdo, Z. Chen, C. Citro, G. S. Corrado, A. Davis, J. Dean, M. Devin, S. Ghemawat, I. Goodfellow, A. Harp, G. Irving, M. Isard, Y. Jia, R. Jozefowicz, L. Kaiser, M. Kudlur, J. Levenberg, D. Mané, R. Monga, S. Moore, D. Murray, C. Olah, M. Schuster, J. Shlens, B. Steiner, I. Sutskever, K. Talwar, P. Tucker, V. Vanhoucke, V. Vasudevan, F. Viégas, O. Vinyals, P. Warden, M. Wattenberg, M. Wicke, Y. Yu, and X. Zheng, "Tensorflow: A

System for Large-Scale Machine Learning," in: *12th USENIX Symposium on Operating Systems Design and Implementation (OSDI 16)*, 2016, 265–283.

[100] T. Bansal, D. -C. Juan, S. Ravi, and A. McCallum, "A2N: Attending to Neighbors for Knowledge Graph Inference," in: *Proceedings of the 57th Annual Meeting of the Association for Computational Linguistics*; Association for Computational Linguistics, 2019.

[101] T. D. Bui, S. Ravi, and V. Ramavajjala, "Neural Graph Learning: Training Neural Networks Using Graphs," in: *Proceedings of the Eleventh ACM International Conference on Web Search and Data Mining*,2018, pp. 64–71.

[102] I. Goodfellow, J. Shlens, and C. Szegedy, "Explaining and Harnessing Adversarial Examples," in: *International Conference on Learning Representations*, 2015.

[103] A. Madry, A. Makelov, L. Schmidt, D. Tsipras, and A. Vladu, Towards Deep Learning Models Resistant to Adversarial Attacks, 2017, arXiv preprint, arXiv:1706.06083.

[104] T. Miyato, S. -I. Maeda, M. Koyama, and S. Ishii, "Virtual Adversarial Training: A Regularization Method for Supervised and Semi-Supervised Learning," In: *IEEE Transactions on Pattern Analysis and Machine Intelligence*, 2019, pp. 1979–1993.

[105] W. Zonghan, S. Pan, F. Chen, G. Long, C. Zhang, and S. Y. Philip, "A Comprehensive Survey on Graph Neural Networks," In: *IEEE Transactions on Neural Networks and Learning Systems*, 2020, pp. 1–21.

[106] R. B. Palm, *Prediction as a Candidate for Learning Deep Hierarchical Models of Data*, 2012.

[107] P. Szymak, P. Piskur, and K. Naus, "The Effectiveness of Using a Pretrained Deep Learning Neural Networks for Object Classification in Underwater Video," *Remote Sensing*, vol. 12, no. 18, p. 3020, 2020, https://doi.org/10.3390/rs12183020

[108] A. Dosovitskiy, L. Beyer, A. Kolesnikov, D. Weissenborn, X. Zhai, T. Unterthiner, M. Dehghani, M. Minderer, G. Heigold, S. Gelly, J. Uszkoreit, and N. Houlsby, "An Image is 11 Worth 16x16 Words: Transformers for Image Recognition at Scale," In *International Conference on Learning Representations*, 2021.

[109] Z. Liu, et al., "Swin Transformer: Hierarchical Vision Transformer using Shifted Windows," In: *2021 IEEE/CVF International Conference on Computer Vision (ICCV)*, 2021, pp. 9992–10002, doi: 10.1109/ICCV48922.2021.00986

[110] Z. Liu, H. Mao, C. -Y. Wu, C. Feichtenhofer, T. Darrell, and S. Xie, "A ConvNet for the 2020s," *CoRR*, т. abs/2201.03545, 2022, https://arxiv.org/abs/2201.03545

[111] D. Castelvecchi, "Can We Open the Black Box of AI?," *Nature News*, vol. 538, no. 7623, p. 20, 2016.

[112] A. Preece, D. Harborne, D. Braines, R. Tomsett, and S. Chakraborty, Stakeholders in Explainable AI, 2018, arXiv:1810.00184.

[113] D. Gunning, Explainable artificial intelligence (xAI), Technical Report, Defense Advanced Research Projects Agency (DARPA), 2017.

[114] E. Tjoa and C. Guan, A Survey on Explainable Artificial Intelligence (XAI): Towards Medical XAI, 2019, arXiv:1907.07374.

[115] J. Zhu, A. Liapis, S. Risi, R. Bidarra, and G. M. Youngblood, "Explainable AI for Designers: A Human-Centered Perspective on Mixed-Initiative Co-creation," in: *2018 IEEE Conference on Computational Intelligence and Games (CIG)*, 2018, pp. 1–8.

[116] M. T. Ribeiro, S. Singh, and C. Guestrin, "Why SHOULD I TRUST YOU?: Explaining the Predictions of Any Classifier," in: *ACM SIGKDD International Conference on Knowledge Discovery and Data Mining*, ACM, 2016, pp. 1135–1144.

[117] M. Fox, D. Long, and D. Magazzeni, Explainable Planning, 2017, arXiv:1709.10256.

[118] H. C. Lane, M. G. Core, M. Van Lent, S. Solomon, and D. Gomboc, Explainable Artificial Intelligence for Training and Tutoring, Technical Report, University of Southern California, 2005.

[119] W. J. Murdoch, C. Singh, K. Kumbier, R. Abbasi-Asl, and B. Yu, "Interpretable Machine Learning: Definitions, Methods, and Applications," 2019, arXiv:1901.04592.

[120] J. Haspiel, N. Du, J. Meyerson, L. P. Robert Jr, D. Tilbury, X. J. Yang, and A. K. Pradhan, "Explanations and Expectations: Trust Building in Automated Vehicles," in: *Companion of the ACM/IEEE International Conference on Human-Robot Interaction*, ACM, 2018, pp. 119–120.

[121] A. Chander, R. Srinivasan, S. Chelian, J. Wang, and K. Uchino, "Working with Beliefs: AI Transparency in the Enterprise," in: *Workshops of the ACM Conference on Intelligent User Interfaces*, 2018.

[122] A. Chouldechova, "Fair Prediction with Disparate Impact: A Study of Bias in Recidivism Prediction Instruments," *Big Data*, vol. 5, no. 2, pp. 153–163, 2017.

[123] M. Kim, O. Reingold, and G. Rothblum, "Fairness Through Computationally-Bounded Awareness," in: *Advances in Neural Information Processing Systems*, 2018, pp. 4842–4852.

[124] S. Tan, R. Caruana, G. Hooker, and Y. Lou, "Distill-and-Compare: Auditing Black-Box Models Using Transparent Model Distillation," in: *AAAI/ACM Conference on AI, Ethics, and Society*, ACM, 2018, pp. 303–310.

[125] R. A. Berk and J. Bleich, "Statistical Procedures for Forecasting Criminal Behavior: A Comparative Assessment," *Criminology & Public Policy*, vol. 12, no. 3, 513–544, 2013.

[126] P. Gajane and M. Pechenizkiy, On Formalizing Fairness in Prediction with Machine Learning, 2017, arXiv:1710.03184.

[127] C. Dwork and C. Ilvento, Composition of Fairsystems, 2018, arXiv:1806.06122.

[128] S. Barocas, M. Hardt, and A. Narayanan, Fairness and Machine Learning, fairmlbook.org, 2019, http://www.fairmlbook.org

[129] K. Burns, L. A. Hendricks, K. Saenko, T. Darrell, and A. Rohrbach, Women also Snowboard: Overcoming Bias in Captioning Models, 2018, arXiv:1803.09797.

[130] A. Bennetot, J.-L. Laurent, R. Chatila, and N. Díaz-Rodríguez, "Towards Explainable Neural-Symbolic Visual Reasoning," in: *NeSy Workshop IJCAI 2019*, Macau, China, 2019.

[131] L. Edwards and M. Veale, "Slave to the Algorithm: Why a Right to an Explanation is Probably not the Remedy You are Looking For," *Duke Law & Technology Review*, vol. 16, p. 18, 2017.

[132] P. Langley, B. Meadows, M. Sridharan, and D. Choi, "Explainable Agency for Intelligent Autonomous Systems," in: *AAAI Conference on Artificial Intelligence*, 2017, pp. 4762–4763.

[133] M. A. Neerincx, J. van der Waa, F. Kaptein, and J. van Diggelen, "Using Perceptual and Cognitive Explanations for Enhanced Human-Agent Team Performance," in: *International Conference on Engineering Psychology and Cognitive Ergonomics*, Springer, 2018, pp. 204–214.

[134] Y. Zhang, S. Sreedharan, A. Kulkarni, T. Chakraborti, H. H. Zhuo, and S. Kambhampati, "Plan Explicability and Predictability for Robot Task Planning," in: *2017 IEEE International Conference on Robotics and Automation (ICRA)*, IEEE, 2017, pp. 1313–1320.

[135] T. Miller, P. Howe, and L. Sonenberg, "Explainable AI: Beware of Inmates Running the Asylum," in: *International Joint Conference on Artificial Intelligence, Workshop on Explainable AI (XAI)*, vol. 36, pp. 36–40, 2017.

[136] H. Hastie, F. J. C. Garcia, D. A. Robb, P. Patron, and A. Laskov, "MIRIAM: A Multimodal Chat-Based Interface for Autonomous Systems," in: *ACM International Conference on Multimodal Interaction*, ACM, 2017, pp. 495–496.

[137] S. Mishra, B. L. Sturm, and S. Dixon, "Local Interpretable Model-Agnostic Explanations for Music Content Analysis," in: *ISMIR*, 2017, pp. 537–543.

[138] M. T. Ribeiro, S. Singh, and C. Guestrin, Nothing Else Matters: Model-Agnostic Explanations by Identifying Prediction Invariance, 2016, arXiv:1611.05817.

[139] U. Johansson, R. König, and L. Niklasson, "The Truth is in There-Rule Extraction from Opaque Models Using Genetic Programming," in: *FLAIRS Conference*, Miami Beach, FL, 2004, pp. 658–663.

[140] U. Johansson, L. Niklasson, and R. König, "Accuracy vs. Comprehensibility in Data Mining Models," in: *Proceedings of the Seventh International Conference on Information Fusion*, vol. 1, pp. 295–300, 2004.

[141] R. Konig, U. Johansson, and L. Niklasson, "G-rex: A Versatile Framework for Evolutionary Data Mining," in: *2008 IEEE International Conference on Data Mining Workshops*, IEEE, 2008, pp. 971–974.

[142] G. Su, D. Wei, K. R. Varshney, and D. M. Malioutov, Interpretable Two-Level Boolean Rule Learning for Classification, 2015, arXiv:1511.07361.

[143] O. Bastani, C. Kim, and H. Bastani, Interpretability via Model Extraction, 2017, arXiv:1706.09773.

[144] P. Cortez and M. J. Embrechts, "Opening Black Box Data Mining Models Using Sensitivity Analysis," in: *2011 IEEE Symposium on Computational Intelligence and Data Mining (CIDM)*, IEEE, 2011, pp. 341–348.

[145] P. Cortez and M. J. Embrechts, "Using Sensitivity Analysis and Visualization Techniques to Open Black Box Data Mining Models," *Information Sciences*, vol. 225, pp. 1–17, 2013.

[146] A. Goldstein, A. Kapelner, J. Bleich, and E. Pitkin, "Peeking Inside the Black Box: Visualizing Statistical Learning with Plots of Individual Conditional Expectation," *Journal of Computational and Graphical Statistics*, vol. 24, no. 1, 44–65, 2015.

[147] S. M. Lundberg and S.-I. Lee, "A Unified Approach to Interpreting Model Predictions," in: *Advances in Neural Information Processing Systems*, 2017, pp. 4765–4774.

[148] I. Kononenko, et al., "An Efficient Explanation of Individual Classifications Using Game Theory," *Journal of Machine Learning Research*, vol. 11, no. Jan, p. 1–18, 2010.

[149] M. Robnik-Šikonja and I. Kononenko, "Explaining Classifications for Individual Instances," *IEEE Transactions on Knowledge and Data Engineering*, vol. 20, no. 5, pp. 589–600, 2008.

[150] D. Baehrens, T. Schroeter, S. Harmeling, M. Kawanabe, K. Hansen, and K.-R. Müller, "How to Explain Individual Classification Decisions," *Journal of Machine Learning Research*, vol. 11, no. Jun, pp. 1803–1831, 2010.

[151] A. Datta, S. Sen, and Y. Zick, "Algorithmic Transparency via Quantitative Input Influence: Theory and Experiments with Learning Systems," in: *2016 IEEE Symposium on Security and Privacy (SP)*, IEEE, 2016, pp. 598–617.

[152] P. Dabkowski and Y. Gal, "Real Time Image Saliency for Black Box Classifiers," in: *Advances in Neural Information Processing Systems*, 2017, pp. 6967–6976.

[153] A. Henelius, K. Puolamäki, and A. Ukkonen, Interpreting Classifiers Through Attribute Interactions in Datasets, 2017, arXiv:1707.07576.

[154] L. Fröhling and A. Zubiaga, "Feature-Based Detection of Automated Language Models: Tackling GPT-2, GPT-3 and Grover," *PeerJ Computer Science*, vol. 7, p. e443, 2021.

## CHAPTER 5

Behavior and Health Status Recognition

5.1 WEARABLE SENSOR-BASED BEHAVIOUR RECOGNITION

As a result of its practical applications, such as innovative healthcare systems, human healthcare derived from body sensor data has received considerable research attention from a wide range of human–computer interaction and pattern analysis researchers in recent wearable sensors-based behavior recognition systems may be used for example, in intelligent clinics to improve the rehabilitation process for patients and extend their independence. The use of distinctive sensors for monitoring vital signs and physical behavior of individuals can be accomplished in many ways; however, physical human activity recognition based on body sensors provides valuable information regarding an individual's lifestyle and functionality [1–26].

Different wearable sensor-based datasets are explored here with machine learning algorithms for different behavior recognition. The datasets for the experiments are publicly available for downloading. This section shows experimental results on other publicly available datasets with codes followed by an example of real-time wearable sensor-based activity recognition.

5.1.1 Mobile Health Dataset and Application

The mobile health (or MHEALTH) public dataset is first considered for feature analysis and activity recognition [12]. The body sensors are placed on the user's body, as shown in Figure 5.1.

As part of the system, sensors are attached to the chest, right wrist, and left ankle. An ECG healthcare sensor, which uses two leads to measure heart data, is connected to the chest. Other sensors are related to motion data. For example, accelerometers are used to measure body acceleration, gyroscopes are used to measure turn rate, and magnetometers

DOI: 10.1201/9781003425908-5

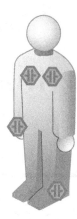

FIGURE 5.1   A user with sensors according to the MHEALTH dataset.

are used to measure magnetic field orientation. As a result of the body sensor data, the following representation can be used:

$$A_C = \left(A_x, A_y, A_z \right).$$

The accelerometer data in the right wrist can be represented as

$$A_{RW} = \left(I_x, I_y, I_z \right).$$

The accelerometer data in the left ankle can be represented as

$$A_{LA} = \left(L_x, L_y, L_z \right).$$

ECG sensor data in the chest can be represented as

$$C = \left(g_1, g_2 \right)$$

The gyroscope sensor data in the left-ankle can be represented as

$$G_{LA} = \left(R_x, R_y, R_z \right).$$

The magnetometer data in the left ankle can be represented as

$$M_{LA} = \left(T_x, T_y, T_z \right).$$

The gyroscope sensor data from the left wrist can be represented as

$$G_{LW} = \left(S_x, S_y, S_z \right).$$

The gyroscope sensor data from the right wrist can be represented as

$$G_{RW} = \left(W_x, W_y, W_z \right).$$

The magnetometer data in the right wrist can be represented as

$$M_{RW} = \left(E_x, E_y, E_z \right).$$

To apply to further machine learning algorithms, the above features are augmented together. First, we collected the MHEALTH dataset to apply the proposed approach and other conventional methods. During 12 different physical activities, 10 subjects were required to record physiological vital signs and body movements. The exercises include standing still, sitting and relaxing, lying down, walking, climbing stairs, bending the waist forward, raising the arms on the front, bending the knees, cycling, jogging, running, and jumping forward and backward. An ECG sensor, an accelerometer, a gyroscope, and a magnetometer were placed on the subject's chest, right wrist, and left ankle to collect the database. Multiple sensors permit the measurement of vital signs, including heart signals using two ECG sensors, acceleration by means of accelerometers, turn rate by means of gyroscopes, and magnetic field orientation by means of magnetometers. A sampling rate of 50 Hz was used to record the sensor modalities.

```python
import numpy as np
import pandas as pd
import seaborn as sns
import matplotlib.pyplot as plt
import tensorflow as tf
from tensorflow.keras.models import Sequential
from tensorflow.keras.layers import Dense
from tensorflow.keras.layers import LSTM
from tensorflow.keras.layers import Embedding

df = pd.read_csv('./mhealth_raw_data.csv')
data = df[df['subject']=='subject2']

for i in range(0,13):

    plt.figure(figsize=(16,4))


    plt.subplot(1,2,1)

    plt.plot(data[ data['Activity']==i ].reset_index(drop=True)['alx'],
alpha=.7, label='Acceleration-lx')

    plt.plot(data[ data['Activity']==i ].reset_index(drop=True)
['aly'],color='green', alpha=.7, label=metric+'Acceleration-ly')

    plt.plot(data[ data['Activity']==i ].reset_index(drop=True)
['alz'],color='red', alpha=.7, label=metric+'Acceleration-lz')
```

```
plt.title(f'{label _ map[i]} - Left-Ankle-Sensor')

plt.legend()


plt.subplot(1,2,2)

plt.plot(data[ data['Activity']==i ].reset _ index(drop=True)['arx'],
alpha=.7, label=metric+'Acceleration-rx')

plt.plot(data[ data['Activity']==i ].reset _ index(drop=True)
['ary'],color='green', alpha=.7, label=metric+'Acceleration-ry')

plt.plot(data[ data['Activity']==i ].reset _ index(drop=True)
['arz'],color='red', alpha=.7, label=metric+'Acceleration-rz')

plt.title(f'{label _ map[i]} - Right-Arm-Sensor')

plt.legend()

plt.show()
```

Figures 5.2–5.14 shows the result of above code where we can see different acceleometer data for different activities where it can be noticed that different acitivities have different distribution.

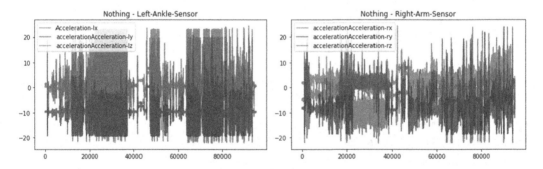

FIGURE 5.2   Left ankle and right arm sensor data of nothing activity from subject 2 of MHEALTH dataset.

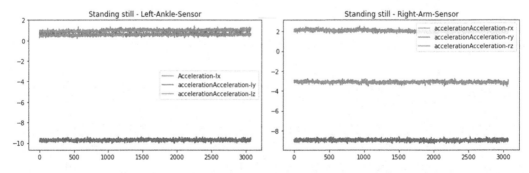

FIGURE 5.3   Left ankle and right arm sensor data of standing activity from subject 2 of MHEALTH dataset.

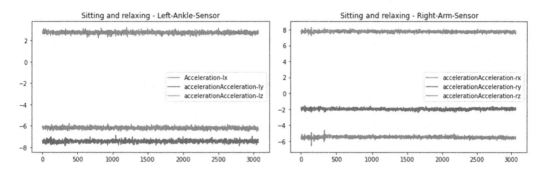

FIGURE 5.4   Left ankle and right arm sensor data of sitting activity from subject 2 of MHEALTH dataset.

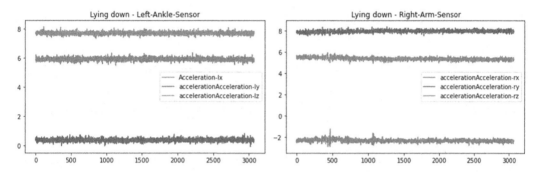

FIGURE 5.5   Left ankle and right arm sensor data of lying down activity from subject 2 of MHEALTH dataset.

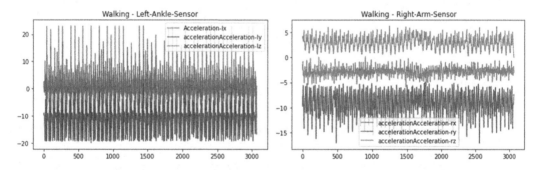

FIGURE 5.6   Left ankle and right arm sensor data of walking activity from subject 2 of MHEALTH dataset.

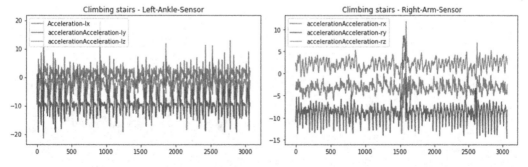

FIGURE 5.7   Left ankle and right arm sensor data of climbing down activity from subject 2 of MHEALTH dataset.

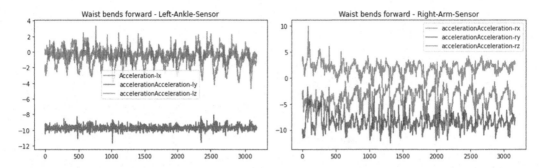

FIGURE 5.8   Left ankle and right arm sensor data of waist bends forward activity from subject 2 of MHEALTH dataset.

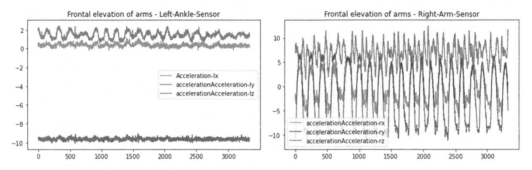

FIGURE 5.9   Left ankle and right arm sensor data of frontal elevation activity from subject 2 of MHEALTH dataset.

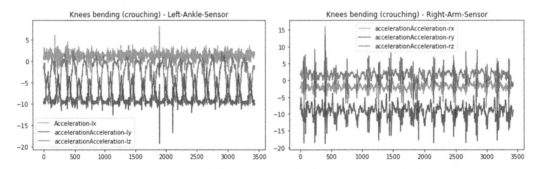

FIGURE 5.10   Left ankle and right arm sensor data of knees bending activity from subject 2 of MHEALTH dataset.

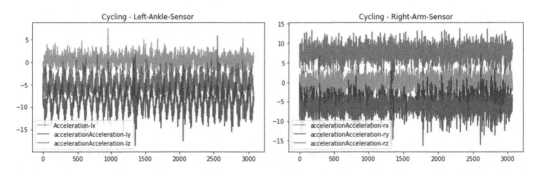

FIGURE 5.11   Left ankle and right arm sensor data of cycling activity from subject 2 of MHEALTH dataset.

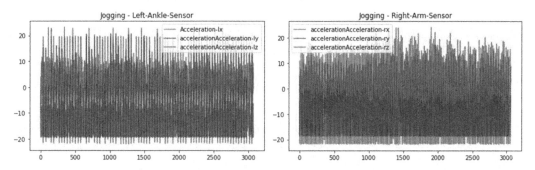

FIGURE 5.12   Left ankle and right arm sensor data of jogging activity from subject 2 of MHEALTH dataset.

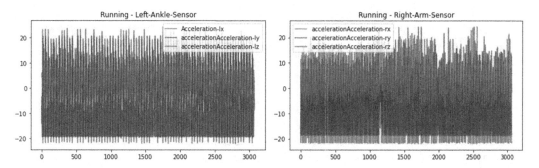

FIGURE 5.13   Left ankle and right arm sensor data of running activity from subject 2 of MHEALTH dataset.

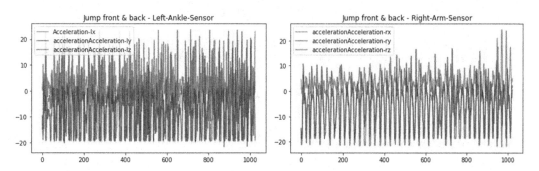

FIGURE 5.14   Left ankle and right arm sensor data of jump front and back activity from subject 2 of MHEALTH dataset.

Now, let us continue the code and see what happens for different experiments as follows:

```
label _ map = {
0: 'Nothing',
1: 'Standing still',
2: 'Sitting and relaxing',
3: 'Lying down',
4: 'Walking',
5: 'Climbing stairs',
6: 'Waist bends forward',
7: 'Frontal elevation of arms',
```

```
8: 'Knees bending (crouching)',
9: 'Cycling',
10: 'Jogging',
11: 'Running',
12: 'Jump front & back'
}

#spliting data into train and test set
train = df[(df['subject'] != 'subject10') & (df['subject'] !=
'subject9')]
test = df.drop(train.index, axis=0)


X _ train = train.drop(['Activity','subject'],axis=1)
y_train = train['Activity']
X_test = test.drop(['Activity','subject'],axis=1)
y_test = test['Activity']

from scipy import stats

#function to create time series dataset for sequence modeling
def create_dataset(X, y, time_steps, step=1):
    Xs, ys = [], []
    for i in range(0, len(X) - time_steps, step):
        x = X.iloc[i:(i + time_steps)].values
        labels = y.iloc[i: i + time_steps]
        Xs.append(x)
        ys.append(stats.mode(labels)[0][0])
    return np.array(Xs), np.array(ys).reshape(-1, 1)

X_train,y_train = create_dataset(X_train, y_train, 100, step=50)
X_train.shape, y_train.shape

X _ test,y _ test = create _ dataset(X _ test, y _ test, 100, step=50)
X_test.shape, y_test.shape

#LSTM
model = Sequential()
model.add(layers.Input(shape=[100,12]))
model.add(layers.LSTM(64))
model.add(layers.Dense(units=128, activation='relu'))
model.add(layers.Dense(13, activation='softmax'))
model.summary()

from sklearn.preprocessing import LabelEncoder
from sklearn.model_selection import train_test_split
from sklearn.metrics import classification_report, accuracy_
score, recall_score, precision_score, f1_score,confusion_
matrix, mean_absolute_error , r2_score , mean_squared_error,
mean_absolute_percentage_error
```

```
tf.keras.utils.plot _ model(model, show _ shapes=True)
tf.keras.utils.plot_model(model1, show_shapes=True)

model.compile(optimizer="adam", loss="sparse _ categorical _
crossentropy", metrics=["sparse _ categorical _ accuracy"],)

model _ history = model.fit(X _ train,y _ train, epochs= 10,
validation _ data=(X _ test,y _ test))

train _ loss = model _ history.history['loss']
val_loss = model_history.history['val_loss']
train_accuracy = model_history.
history['sparse_categorical_accuracy']
val_accuracy = model_history.
history['val_sparse_categorical_accuracy']

train _ loss, train _ acc = model.evaluate(X _ train,y _ train)
test_loss, test_acc = model.evaluate(X_test,y_test)

print("Train accuracy", round(train _ acc*100, 2),'%')
print("Train loss", train_loss)
print("Test accuracy", round(test_acc*100, 2),'%')
print("Test loss", test_loss)

plt.figure(figsize=(12,6))

plt.subplot(1,2,1)
plt.plot(train_loss, 'r', label='Training loss')
plt.plot(val_loss, 'b', label='Validation loss')
plt.title('Training and Validation Loss')
plt.xlabel('Epoch')
plt.ylabel('Loss Value')
plt.legend()
plt.show()

pred = model.predict(X _ test)
pred = np.argmax(pred, axis = 1)
pred = pred.reshape(-1,1)
classes = ['Nothing', 'Standing still', 'Sitting and relaxing',
'Lying down', 'Walking', 'Climbing stairs', 'Waist bends
forward', 'Frontal elevation of arms',
          'Knees bending (crouching)', 'Cycling', 'Jogging',
'Running', 'Jump front & back']

data _ columns=list(train.columns)
data_columns =data_columns[0:12]
```

```python
from lime import lime _ tabular
explainer = lime_tabular.RecurrentTabularExplainer(X_train,
training_labels=y_train, feature_names=data_columns,
                                discretize_continuous=True,
                                class_names=classes,
                                discretizer='decile')

exp = explainer.explain _ instance(X _ test[[0],:,:], model.predict,
num _ features=12, labels=(1,))
exp.show_in_notebook()

p = model.predict(X _ test[[0],:,:])
p = np.argmax(p, axis = 1)
print(p)


from sklearn.metrics import confusion_matrix,
classification_report

print(classification _ report(y _ test,pred))
print('*'*50)
print(confusion_matrix(y_test,pred))

plt.figure(figsize=(12,8))
conf_matrix = confusion_matrix(y_test,pred)
sns.heat sns.heatmap(conf_matrix, annot=True, fmt='.2f',
cmap='Blues')
plt.show()

cmn = conf _ matrix.astype('float') / conf _ matrix.sum(axis=1)[:,
np.newaxis]
fig, ax = plt.subplots(figsize=(10,10))
sns.heatmap(cmn, annot=True, fmt='.2f', cmap='Blues')
plt.ylabel('Actual')
plt.xlabel('Predicted')
plt.show(block=False)
#NSL
h,w,l=X_train.shape
model = tf.keras.Sequential([
        tf.keras.Input((w, l), name='feature'),
        tf.keras.layers.Flatten(),
        tf.keras.layers.Dense(128, activation=tf.nn.relu),
        tf.keras.layers.Dense(64, activation=tf.nn.relu),
        tf.keras.layers.Dense(13, activation=tf.nn.softmax)
        ])

import tensorflow as tf
import neural_structured_learning as nsl
```

```
adv _ config = nsl.configs.make _ adv _ reg _ config(multiplier=0.1,
adv _ step _ size=0.1)
adv_model = nsl.keras.AdversarialRegularization(model,
adv_config=adv_config)
 # Compile, train, and evaluate.
adv_model.compile(optimizer='adam',loss='sparse_categorical_
crossentropy', metrics=['accuracy'])
adv_model.fit({'feature': X_train, 'label': y_train}, batch_
size=20, epochs=100, verbose=0)
scores = adv_model.evaluate({'feature': X_test, 'label': y_test},
verbose=0)
print("%.2f%%" % scores[2])


from tensorflow.keras.utils import to _ categorical
y_train = to_categorical(y_train, dtype ="uint8")
y_test = to_categorical(y_test, dtype ="uint8")


#CNN


model _ cnn = Sequential()
model_cnn.add(layers.Conv1D(filters=64, kernel_size=3,
activation='relu', input_shape=(100,12)))
model_cnn.add(layers.Conv1D(filters=64, kernel_size=3,
activation='relu'))
model_cnn.add(layers.Dropout(0.5))
model_cnn.add(layers.MaxPooling1D(pool_size=2))
model_cnn.add(layers.Flatten())
model_cnn.add(layers.Dense(100, activation='relu'))
model_cnn.add(layers.Dense(13, activation='softmax'))
model_cnn.summary()

model _ cnn.compile(loss='categorical _ crossentropy',
optimizer='adam', metrics=['accuracy'])


model _ cnn _ history = model _ cnn.fit(X _ train,y _ train, epochs=
100, validation _ data=(X _ test,y _ test))
test_loss, test_acc_cnn = model_cnn.evaluate(X_test,y_test)
                                    print(test_acc_cnn)
```

Figures 5.15 and 5.16 shows the confusion matrix based on number of samples and normalized samples, respectively using LSTM. Figure 5.17 shows the epoch versus model loss using LSTM model. Figure 5.18 shows an explanation of a test sample using LIME. The results are shown using above code. Also, above code shows how to implement NSL and CNN on the same dataset, indicating efforts to try distinguished models to compare.

	0	1	2	3	4	5	6	7	8	9	10	11	12
0	2470	139	0	47	96	22	6	35	21	18	19	5	12
1	122	0	0	0	0	0	0	0	0	0	0	0	0
2	122	0	0	0	0	0	0	0	0	0	0	0	0
3	0	0	0	122	0	0	0	0	0	0	0	0	0
4	57	0	0	0	62	0	0	0	0	0	0	0	0
5	3	0	0	0	0	90	0	0	0	0	0	0	0
6	98	0	0	0	0	0	8	0	0	0	0	0	0
7	22	0	0	0	0	0	0	91	0	0	0	0	0
8	32	0	0	0	0	0	0	0	84	0	0	0	0
9	8	0	0	0	0	0	0	0	0	109	0	0	0
10	10	0	0	0	0	0	0	0	0	0	69	0	0
11	5	0	0	0	0	0	0	0	0	0	2	22	0
12	5	0	0	0	0	0	0	0	0	0	0	0	15

FIGURE 5.15   Confusion matrix of 12 activities from MHEALTH dataset.

Table 5.1 shows experimental results from different approaches where NSL shows highest mean accuracy. This result may vary using different parameters of the model and training time.

5.1.2 PUC-Rio Dataset

We examined the PUC-Rio behavior recognition dataset [15] as our second body sensor database. This dataset was recorded using accelerometers placed at four different points on the body, namely the waist, left thigh, right ankle, and right arm. The sensor placement is shown in Figure 5.19. Before the data collection process, the accelerometer sensors were calibrated. During the calibration process, the sensors were positioned and the sensor values were read. In order to reduce the read parameters obtained at the beginning of the calibration process from the values obtained at the time of the calibration, the read parameters were subtracted from the values obtained at the beginning of the data-processing process. For the purpose of maintaining a high standard of data collection, the body sensors were mounted on top of a flat table at the same position, and calibration was performed

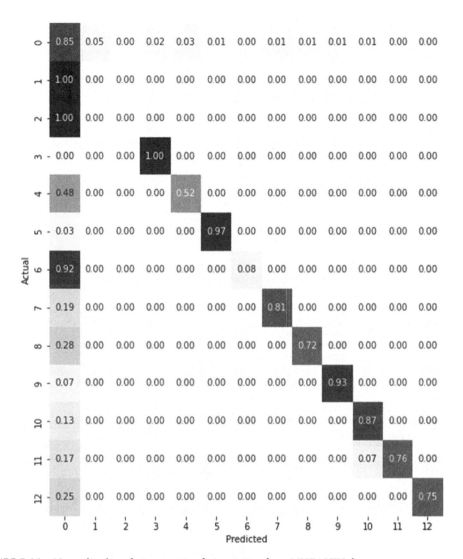

FIGURE 5.16   Normalized confusion matrix of 12 activities from MHEALTH dataset.

thereafter. In the second type of calibration, the accelerometers were calibrated against the subjects, and the data was read after placing the sensors at the same places on their bodies.

The sensor data are represented as follows. The accelerometer data in waist can be represented as

$$C_w = \left(A_x, A_y, A_z\right).$$

The accelerometer data in the left thigh can be represented as

$$C_{LT} = \left(L_x, L_y, L_z\right).$$

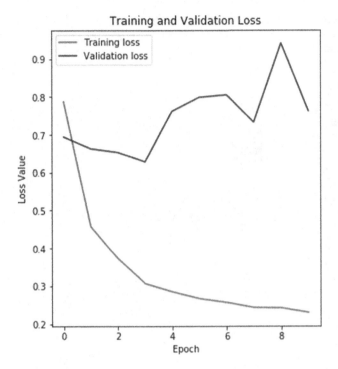

FIGURE 5.17 Loss versus epochs of training and validation of LSTM model on MHEALTH dataset.

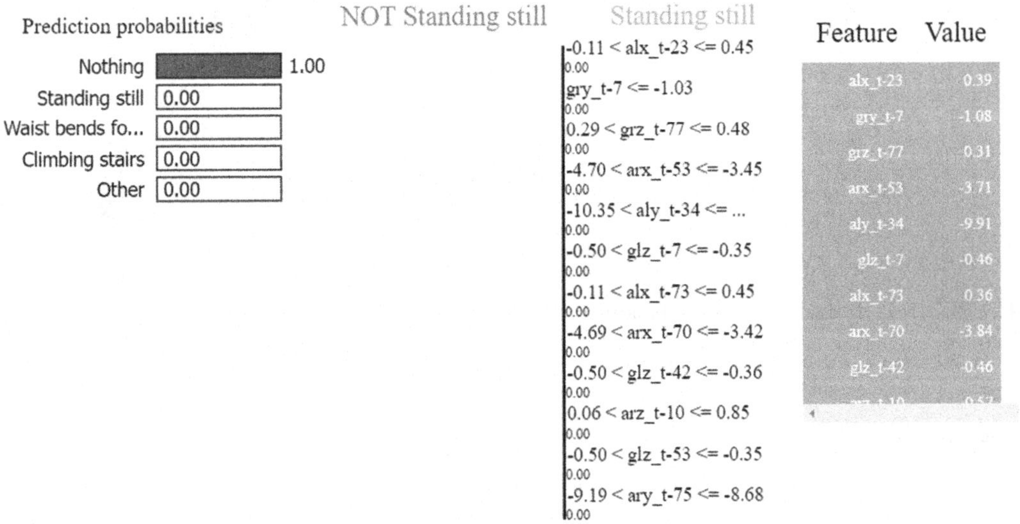

FIGURE 5.18 Explanation of test sample using LIME on LSTM model.

The accelerometer data in the right ankle can be represented as

$$W_{RA} = (W_x, W_y, W_z).$$

The accelerometer data in the right upper arm be represented as

$$C_{RA} = (R_x, R_y, R_z).$$

TABLE 5.1   The Accuracies of Different Activities Using Different
Approaches on MHEALTH Dataset

Activity#	Activity/model	CNN	LSTM	NSL
0	Standing still	1.00	1.00	1.00
1	Sitting and relaxing	0.90	0.92	1.00
2	Lying down	0.85	0.91	0.99
3	Walking	1.00	1.00	1.00
4	Climbing stairs	0.91	0.94	0.99
5	Waist bends forward	0.93	1.00	1.00
6	Frontal elevation of arms	0.94	0.90	1.00
7	Knees bending	0.89	0.92	1.00
8	Cycling	0.90	1.00	1.00
9	Jogging	0.92	0.91	0.99
10	Running	0.92	0.97	0.99
11	Jump front and back	0.89	0.92	1.00
	Mean	**0.92**	**0.94**	**0.99**

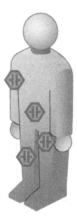

FIGURE 5.19   A user wearing sensor on body according to PUC-Rio dataset.

Furthermore, other statistical features, such as mean, variance, standard deviation, and skewness, are extracted from the data, and fusion is done to augment them with other features. All the features are usually augmented to further apply on deep learning models.

There are five different activities included in the dataset PUC-Rio Dataset. There are 165,632 samples in the dataset for the five activities, namely sitting, sitting down, standing, standing up, and walking. The dataset has a total of 165,632 samples. A two-fold cross-validation was conducted there. The following sample code shows the similar example as done before for MHEALTH dataset. Figures 5.20 and 5.21 show the model convergence plot and XAI results using LIME, respectively. Table 5.2 shows different results using different approaches on the dataset where LSTM shows highest mean accuracy.

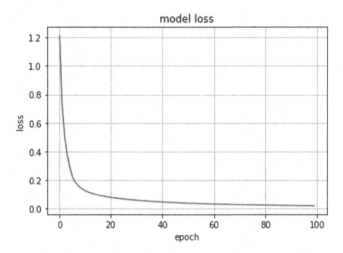

FIGURE 5.20   Model loss versus epochs of LSTM model on PUC-Rio dataset.

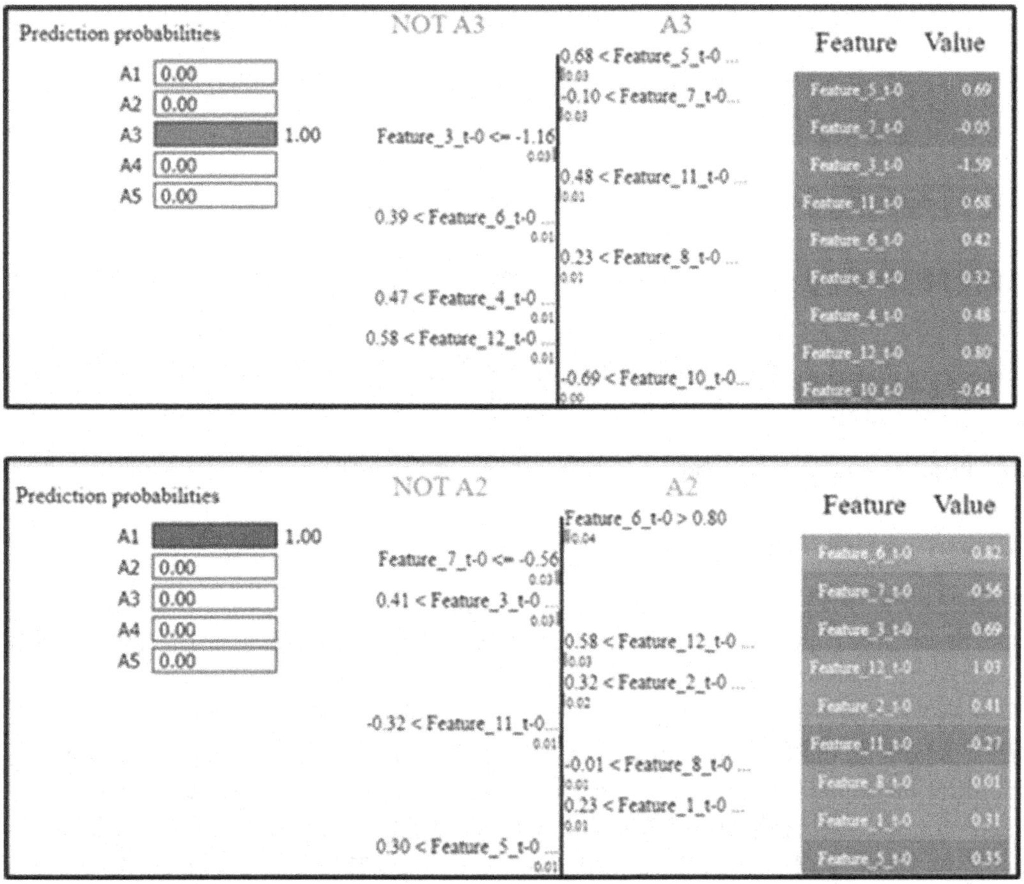

FIGURE 5.21   Two examples of feature importance using LIME on LSTM model of PUC-Rio dataset.

TABLE 5.2   The Accuracies of Different Activities Using Different Approaches

Activity/model	CNN	NSL	LSTM
Sitting	1.00	1.00	1.00
Sitting Down	0.90	0.92	0.98
Standing	0.85	0.91	1.00
Standing Up	1.00	1.00	0.97
Walking	0.91	0.94	0.99
Mean	**0.92**	**0.94**	**0.99**

```
import scipy.io
import numpy as np
from tensorflow.keras.datasets import imdb
from tensorflow.keras.models import Sequential
from tensorflow.keras.layers import Dense
from tensorflow.keras.layers import LSTM
from tensorflow.keras.preprocessing import sequence
# fix random seed for reproducibility

data _ dim = 12
timesteps = 1
num_classes = 5

# expected input data shape: (batch _ size, timesteps, data _ dim)
model = Sequential()
model.add(LSTM(50, return_sequences=True,
               input_shape=(timesteps, data_dim)))  # returns a
sequence of vectors of dimension 32
model.add(LSTM(50))  # return a single vector of dimension 32
model.add(Dense(5, activation='softmax'))

model.compile(loss='categorical _ crossentropy',
              optimizer='rmsprop',
              metrics=['accuracy'])

matData = scipy.io.loadmat('./data _ fold1.mat')
X_train = matData['train_x']
X_test = matData['test_x']
Y_train = matData['train_y']
Y_test = matData['test_y']

X _ train=np.reshape(X _ train, (82816, 1, 12))
X_test=np.reshape(X_test, (82817, 1, 12))
y_train=np.reshape(Y_train, (82816,5))
y_test=np.reshape(Y_test, (82817, 5))

#model.summary()
history=model.fit(x_train, y_train, epochs=100, batch_size=1000)
import scipy.io
import numpy as np
from tensorflow.keras.datasets import imdb
```

```
from tensorflow.keras.models import Sequential
from tensorflow.keras.layers import Dense
from tensorflow.keras.layers import LSTM
from tensorflow.keras.preprocessing import sequence
# fix random seed for reproducibility

data _ dim = 12
timesteps = 1
num_classes = 5

# expected input data shape: (batch _ size, timesteps, data _ dim)
model = Sequential()
model.add(LSTM(50, return_sequences=True, f
              input_shape=(timesteps, data_dim)))  # returns a
sequence of vectors of dimension 32
model.add(LSTM(50))  # return a single vector of dimension 32
model.add(Dense(5, activation='softmax'))

model.compile(loss='categorical _ crossentropy',
              optimizer='rmsprop',
              metrics=['accuracy'])

matData = scipy.io.loadmat('./data _ fold1.mat')
X_train = matData['train_x']
X_test = matData['test_x']
Y_train = matData['train_y']
Y_test = matData['test_y']

X _ train=np.reshape(X _ train, (82816, 1, 12))
X_test=np.reshape(X_test, (82817, 1, 12))
y_train=np.reshape(Y_train, (82816,5))
y_test=np.reshape(Y_test, (82817, 5))

#model.summary()
history=model.fit(x_train, y_train, epochs=100, batch_size=1000)
score, acc = model.evaluate(X_test, y_test,
                            batch_size=1000)
print('Test score:', score)
print('Test accuracy:', acc)

import matplotlib.pyplot as plt

# "Loss"
plt.plot(history.history['loss'])
plt.title('model loss')
plt.ylabel('loss')
plt.xlabel('epoch')

plt.grid()

#plt.legend(['train', 'validation'], loc='upper left')
plt.show()
```

```
data_columns = [ 'Feature_{}'.format(x) for x in range(1,13)]
from lime import lime_tabular

explainer = lime_tabular.RecurrentTabularExplainer(X_train,
training_labels=y_train, feature_names=data_columns,
                    discretize_continuous=True,
                    class_names=['A1', 'A2','A3', 'A4','A5' ],
                    discretizer='decile')
exp = explainer.explain_instance(X_test[100], model.predict, num_
features=10, labels=(1,))
exp.show_in_notebook()
exp = explainer.explain_instance(X_test[54001], model.predict,
num_features=10, labels=(2,))
exp.show_in_notebook()
```

5.1.3 ARem Dataset

The third dataset to apply the proposed approach that we choose is Activity Recognition system based on Multisensor data fusion (AReM) dataset [16]. The dataset serves as a benchmark in activity analysis applications where the activity recognition is based on time-series data collected by a Wireless Sensor Network. Information is used that is derived from implicit changes in the wireless channel resulting from the motion of the user in the dataset. During the exchange of beacon packets within sensor networks, the sensor devices measure the received signal strength (RSS). As shown in Figure 5.22, users wear chest and ankle sensors. The raw data is slightly noise-removed. An epoch time of 250 milliseconds is selected in the dataset, which allows for the collection of five RSS samples for each of the three couples of body sensor nodes within that period. This dataset contains the mean and variance of the RSS values obtained from the three sensor pairs.

The sensor features are augmented as follows:

$$F_{\text{AReM}} = \left(mean\_rss12, var\_rss12, mean\_rss13, \ var\_rss13, mean\_rss23, var\_rss23 \right).$$

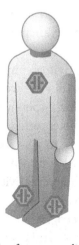

FIGURE 5.22   Sensor placements on the body of user according to AReM dataset.

TABLE 5.3   Accuracies of Different Activities Using Different
Approaches on AReM Dataset

Activity/Model	DBN	CNN	LSTM	NSL
Walking	0.92	1.00	1.00	1.00
Standing	0.91	0.90	0.92	1.00
Sitting	0.84	0.85	0.91	0.99
Lying	0.92	1.00	1.00	1.00
Cycling	0.93	0.91	0.94	0.99
Bending	0.90	0.93	1.00	1.00
Mean	**0.90**	**0.92**	**0.94**	0.99

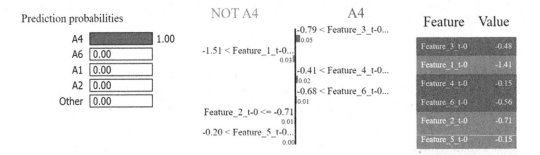

FIGURE 5.23   Feature importance using LIME on LSTM model of AreM dataset.

AReM dataset was developed after conducting experiments on two public datasets. For the training and testing, we chose a random split of the number of samples. We considered six activities from the dataset: walking, standing, sitting, lying, cycling, and bending. Similar example code to that used in the previous experiments stated before can be applied on this dataset as well. Table 5.3 shows the results of various approaches using LSTM-based approaches, where the LSTM-based approach achieved the highest mean recall rates. Figure 5.23 shows a LIME example of how to explain feature importance using the NSL-trained model.

5.1.4 WISDM Dataset

The WISDM (Wireless Sensor Data Mining) Smartphone and Smartwatch Activity and Biometrics Dataset play a crucial role in advancing sensor data analysis, wearable technology, and health monitoring. This dataset is a goldmine for researchers and developers, providing valuable insights into human activities, physiological responses, and the complex relationship between our actions and the devices we wear. At its heart, the WISDM dataset is a compilation of data collected from smartphones and smartwatches, both armed with an array of sensors, including accelerometers and gyroscopes. This gathering process captures a diverse array of activities, aiming to give a comprehensive understanding of how these devices react to various movements and scenarios in real-world situations.

The dataset spans a wide spectrum of human activities, from the everyday, like walking and sitting, to more dynamic actions such as jogging or climbing stairs. This inclusivity makes WISDM a robust resource for activity recognition research, a critical aspect in applications like fitness tracking, healthcare monitoring, and context-aware computing. One notable feature of WISDM is its integration of biometric data alongside traditional sensor readings.

Beyond tracking physical activities, the dataset includes information about heart rate and other physiological parameters. This fusion of multimodal data allows researchers to explore the correlation between our physical endeavors and the body's responses. It not only enriches the dataset but also caters to a broader spectrum of research interests, from pure activity recognition to the intricate interplay of physical exertion and health metrics. The significance of the WISDM dataset resonates across multiple domains. In the field of activity recognition, researchers leverage this dataset to develop and refine algorithms capable of accurately classifying various physical activities. These algorithms find practical applications in fitness monitoring, sports analytics, and healthcare, where understanding and quantifying human movement are pivotal. Furthermore, the inclusion of biometric data extends the utility of WISDM into health and wellness research. The dataset becomes a playground for exploring how different activities impact our physiological well-being. Real-time monitoring of heart rate during exercise or daily activities contributes to the development of health-centric applications, empowering individuals to track and improve their well-being. The world of wearable technology, always at the forefront of innovation, significantly benefits from datasets like WISDM. It provides real-world sensor data that aids in the development and testing of algorithms for smartwatches and smartphones. Wearable device manufacturers use such datasets to optimize sensor performance, ensuring these devices accurately capture and interpret user activities. The dataset's relevance extends into the human–computer interaction (HCI) field. Understanding how users interact with devices in real-world scenarios is crucial for creating intelligent and responsive systems. WISDM's dataset, with its diverse set of activities and biometric readings, provides a realistic foundation for developing systems that adapt to users' behaviours and needs. As with any dataset, there are challenges and considerations accompanying the use of WISDM. Privacy concerns loom large, given the personal nature of the data collected. Researchers and developers must navigate ethical guidelines and privacy regulations to ensure the responsible use of such sensitive information.

The dataset comprises information gathered from 34 individuals, each tasked with performing 18 activities of 3 minutes' duration. Participants wore a smartwatch on their dominant hand and carried a smartphone in their pocket as shown in Figure 5.24. A custom app, operating on both the smartphone and smartwatch, orchestrated the data

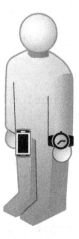

FIGURE 5.24   A user carrying a smartphone and smartwatch used for WISDM dataset.

TABLE 5.4   Activities and Codes from WISDM Dataset

Activity	Code
Walking	A
Jogging	B
Stairs	C
Sitting	D
Standing	E
Typing	F
Brushing Teeth	G
Eating Soup	H
Eating Chips	I
Eating Pasta	J
Drinking from Cup	K
Eating Sandwich	L
Kicking (Soccer Ball)	M
Playing Catch w/Tennis Ball	O
Dribbling (Basketball)	P
Writing	Q
Clapping	R
Folding Clothes	S

collection. Four sensors, including accelerometers and gyroscopes on both devices, contributed to the dataset. The data was recorded at a 20 Hz rate, equating to every 50 milliseconds. The smartphones utilized were either the Google Nexus 5/5X or the Samsung Galaxy S5, operating on Android 6.0 (Marshmallow). The LG G Watch, running Android Wear 1.5, served as the smartwatch. The following table shows the activities and corresponding codes. Since the activity list is a bit long, they are expressed in letters, as shown in Table 5.4.

Here is a sample code using LSTM and LIME:

```
import numpy as np
import pandas as pd
import os
for dirname, _, filenames in os.walk('./wisdm-dataset/raw/phone/
accel'):
    for filename in filenames:
        print(os.path.join(dirname, filename))
from __future__ import print_function
from matplotlib import pyplot as plt
get_ipython().run_line_magic('matplotlib', 'inline')
import numpy as np
import pandas as pd
import seaborn as sns
#import coremltools
from scipy import stats
from IPython.display import display, HTML
```

```python
from sklearn import metrics
from sklearn.metrics import classification_report
from sklearn import preprocessing
from tensorflow.keras.models import Sequential
from tensorflow.keras.layers import Dense
from tensorflow.keras.layers import LSTM
from tensorflow.keras.preprocessing import sequence
from keras.utils import np_utils

columns=['user','activity','time','x','y','z']

data _ phone _ accel _ sum = pd.DataFrame(data=None,columns=columns)
for dirname, _, filenames in os.walk('./wisdm-dataset/raw/phone/
accel'):
    for filename in filenames:
        df = pd.read_csv('./wisdm-dataset/raw/phone/
accel/'+filename , sep=",", header=None)
        temp=pd.DataFrame(data=df.values, columns=columns)
        data_phone_accel_sum=pd.
concat([data_phone_accel_sum,temp])

data _ phone _ accel _ sum['z'] = data _ phone _ accel _ sum['z'].str.
replace(';',")
data_phone_accel_sum['activity'].value_counts()
data_phone_accel_sum['x']=data_phone_accel_sum['x'].astype('float')
data_phone_accel_sum['y']=data_phone_accel_sum['y'].astype('float')
data_phone_accel_sum['z']=data_phone_accel_sum['z'].astype('float')
data_phone_accel_sum.info()

# Phone Gyro files import Train/test
data_phone_gyro_sum = pd.DataFrame(data=None,columns=columns)
for dirname, _, filenames in os.walk('./wisdm-dataset/raw/phone/
gyro'):
    for filename in filenames:
        df = pd.read_csv('./wisdm-dataset/raw/phone/
gyro/'+filename , sep=",", header=None)
        temp=pd.DataFrame(data=df.values, columns=columns)
        data_phone_gyro_sum=pd.concat([data_phone_gyro_sum,temp])

data _ phone _ gyro _ sum['z'] = data _ phone _ gyro _ sum['z'].str.
replace(';',")

data_phone_gyro_sum['x']=data_phone_gyro_sum['x'].astype('float')
data_phone_gyro_sum['y']=data_phone_gyro_sum['y'].astype('float')
data_phone_gyro_sum['z']=data_phone_gyro_sum['z'].astype('float')

# Watch Gyro files import train/test

data _ watch _ gyro _ sum = pd.DataFrame(data=None,columns=columns)
for dirname, _, filenames in os.walk('./wisdm-dataset/raw/watch/gyro'):
```

```
        for filename in filenames:
            df = pd.read_csv('./wisdm-dataset/raw/watch/
gyro/'+filename , sep=",", header=None)
            temp=pd.DataFrame(data=df.values, columns=columns)
            data_watch_gyro_sum=pd.concat([data_watch_gyro_sum,temp])

data_watch_gyro_sum['z'] = data_watch_gyro_sum['z'].str.
replace(';',")
data_watch_gyro_sum['x']=data_watch_gyro_sum['x'].astype('float')
data_watch_gyro_sum['y']=data_watch_gyro_sum['y'].astype('float')
data_watch_gyro_sum['z']=data_watch_gyro_sum['z'].astype('float')

# Watch accelerometer files import train test

data _ watch _ accel _ sum = pd.DataFrame(data=None,columns=columns)
for dirname, _, filenames in os.walk('./wisdm-dataset/raw/watch/
accel'):
    for filename in filenames:
        df = pd.read_csv('./wisdm-dataset/raw/watch/
accel/'+filename , sep=",", header=None)
        temp=pd.DataFrame(data=df.values, columns=columns)
        data_watch_accel_sum=pd.
concat([data_watch_accel_sum,temp])

data_watch_accel_sum['z'] = data_watch_accel_sum['z'].str.
replace(';',")
data_watch_accel_sum['x']=data_watch_accel_sum['x'].astype('float')
data_watch_accel_sum['y']=data_watch_accel_sum['y'].astype('float')
data_watch_accel_sum['z']=data_watch_accel_sum['z'].astype('float')

data _ watch _ accel _ sum['activity'].value _ counts()
data_watch_accel_sum.info()

# Combining Phone accel and gyro data
df_phone = pd.DataFrame(data=None, columns=columns)
df_phone['user']= data_phone_accel_sum['user'].head(3608635)
df_phone['activity']= data_phone_accel_sum['activity'].
head(3608635)
df_phone['time']= data_phone_accel_sum['time'].head(3608635)
df_phone['x'] = data_phone_gyro_sum['x'].values + data_phone_
accel_sum['x'].head(3608635).values
df_phone['y'] = data_phone_gyro_sum['y'].values + data_phone_
accel_sum['y'].head(3608635).values
df_phone['z'] = data_phone_gyro_sum['z'].values + data_phone_
accel_sum['z'].head(3608635).values

# Combining watch accel and gyro data
df_watch = pd.DataFrame(data=None, columns=columns)
df_watch['user']= data_watch_accel_sum['user'].head(3440342)
df_watch['activity']= data_watch_accel_sum['activity'].
head(3440342)
```

```
df_watch['time']= data_watch_accel_sum['time'].head(3440342)
df_watch['x'] = data_watch_gyro_sum['x'].values + data_watch_
accel_sum['x'].head(3440342).values
df_watch['y'] = data_watch_gyro_sum['x'].values + data_watch_
accel_sum['y'].head(3440342).values
df_watch['z'] = data_watch_gyro_sum['x'].values + data_watch_
accel_sum['z'].head(3440342).values

# Combining Phone and Watch Data
df_phone_watch = pd.DataFrame(data=None, columns=columns)
df_phone_watch['user']= df_phone['user'].head(3440342)
df_phone_watch['activity']= df_phone['activity'].head(3440342)
df_phone_watch['time']= df_phone['time'].head(3440342)
df_phone_watch['x'] = df_watch['x'].values + df_phone['x'].
head(3440342).values
df_phone_watch['y'] = df_watch['y'].values + df_phone['y'].
head(3440342).values
df_phone_watch['z'] = df_watch['z'].values + df_phone['z'].
head(3440342).values


Fs = 20
activities = df _ phone _ watch['activity'].value _ counts().index
df_phone_watch = df_phone_watch.drop(['user', 'time'], axis=1)

df_a = df_phone_watch[df_phone_watch['activity']=='A'].head(174604)
df_m = df_phone_watch[df_phone_watch['activity']=='M'].head(174604)
df_k = df_phone_watch[df_phone_watch['activity']=='K'].head(174604)
df_p = df_phone_watch[df_phone_watch['activity']=='P'].head(174604)
df_e = df_phone_watch[df_phone_watch['activity']=='E'].head(174604)
df_o = df_phone_watch[df_phone_watch['activity']=='O'].head(174604)
df_c = df_phone_watch[df_phone_watch['activity']=='C'].head(174604)
df_d = df_phone_watch[df_phone_watch['activity']=='D'].head(174604)
df_l = df_phone_watch[df_phone_watch['activity']=='L'].head(174604)
df_b = df_phone_watch[df_phone_watch['activity']=='B'].head(174604)
df_h = df_phone_watch[df_phone_watch['activity']=='H'].head(174604)
df_f = df_phone_watch[df_phone_watch['activity']=='F'].head(174604)
df_g = df_phone_watch[df_phone_watch['activity']=='G'].head(174604)
df_q = df_phone_watch[df_phone_watch['activity']=='Q'].head(174604)
df_r = df_phone_watch[df_phone_watch['activity']=='R'].head(174604)
df_s = df_phone_watch[df_phone_watch['activity']=='S'].head(174604)
df_i = df_phone_watch[df_phone_watch['activity']=='I'].head(174604)
df_j = df_phone_watch[df_phone_watch['activity']=='J']

balanced _ data = pd.DataFrame()
balanced_data = balanced_data.append([df_a,df_m,df_k,df_p,df_e,df_
o,df_c,df_d,df_l,df_b,df_h,df_f,df_g,df_q,df_r,df_s,df_i,df_j])
balanced_data['activity'].value_counts()

from sklearn.preprocessing import LabelEncoder
label = LabelEncoder()
balanced_data['label'] = label.fit_transform(balanced_data['activity'])
```

```python
from sklearn.preprocessing import StandardScaler

x = balanced _ data[['x','y','z']]
y = balanced_data['label']
scaler = StandardScaler()
x = scaler.fit_transform(x)
scaled_x = pd.DataFrame(data=x, columns=['x','y','z'])
scaled_x['label'] = y.values

# **Frame Preparation**
import scipy.stats as stats
Fs=20
frame_size = Fs*4 #80
hop_size = Fs*2 #40

def get _ frames(df, frame _ size, hop _ size):
    N_FEATURES = 3
    frames = []
    labels = []
    for i in range(0,len(df )- frame_size, hop_size):
        x = df['x'].values[i: i+frame_size]
        y = df['y'].values[i: i+frame_size]
        z = df['z'].values[i: i+frame_size]

        label = stats.mode(df['label'][i: i+frame _ size])[0][0]
        frames.append([x,y,z])
        labels.append(label)

    frames = np.asarray(frames).reshape(-1, frame _ size,
N _ FEATURES)
    labels = np.asarray(labels)

    return frames, labels

x,y = get _ frames(scaled _ x, frame _ size, hop _ size)

from sklearn.model _ selection import train _ test _ split
x_train, x_test, y_train, y_test = train_test_split(x,y,test_
size=0.30, random_state = 0, stratify = y)

# create and fit the LSTM network
model = Sequential()
model.add(LSTM(50,  return_sequences=True, input_shape=(80,3)))
model.add(LSTM(20))
model.add(Dense(18))
model.compile(loss='mean_squared_error', optimizer='adam')
history = model.fit(x_train , y_train, epochs=50, batch_size=100,
verbose=1)

import matplotlib.pyplot as plt
```

```python
plt.plot(history.history['loss'], label='train_loss')
#plt.plot(history.history['val_loss'], label='val_loss')
plt.title('Training  Loss')
plt.xlabel('Epoch')
plt.ylabel('Loss')
plt.legend()
plt.show()

import numpy as np
preds = model.predict(x_test)
y_preds = np.argmax(preds , axis = 1 )

#confusion matrix
import seaborn as sns
from sklearn.metrics import confusion_matrix
cm_data = confusion_matrix(y_test , y_preds)
cm = pd.DataFrame(cm_data, columns=label.classes_, index = label.
classes_)
cm.index.name = 'Actual'
cm.columns.name = 'Predicted'
plt.figure(figsize = (20,10))
plt.title('Confusion Matrix', fontsize = 10)
sns.set(font_scale=1.2)
ax = sns.heatmap(cm, cbar=False, cmap="Blues", annot=True, annot_
kws={"size": 16}, fmt='g')

#confusion matrix normalized
cmn = cm_data.astype('float') / cm_data.sum(axis=1)[:, np.newaxis]
cmn = pd.DataFrame(cmn, columns=label.classes_, index = label.
classes_)
cmn.index.name = 'Actual'
cmn.columns.name = 'Predicted'
plt.figure(figsize = (20,10))
plt.title('Confusion Matrix', fontsize = 10)
sns.set(font_scale=1.2)
sns.heatmap(cmn, annot=True, fmt='.2f', cmap="Blues",
xticklabels=label.classes_, yticklabels=label.classes_)

#XAI

import numpy as np
from lime import lime_tabular
data_columns = [ 'Feature_{}'.format(x) for x in range(1,80)]

explainer = lime _ tabular.RecurrentTabularExplainer(x _
train, training _ labels=y _ train, feature _ names=data _
columns,                          discretize _ continuous=True,
class _ names=label.classes _ ,          discretizer='decile')
```

```
exp = explainer.explain_instance(x_test[8], model.predict, num_
features=80, labels=(6,))
exp.show_in_notebook()
```

The code generates following results using LSTM where Figure 5.25 shows model convergence plot, Figure 5.26 confusion matrix based on samples, Figure 5.27 normalized confusion matrix, and Figure 5.28 LIME example.

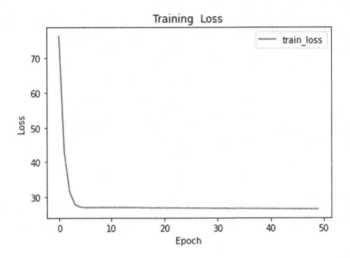

FIGURE 5.25   Epoch versus loss of LSTM model on the WISDM dataset.

Confusion Matrix

	A	B	C	D	E	F	G	H	I	J	K	L	M	O	P	Q	R	S
A	135	61	0	52	56	0	262	148	282	5	2	23	2	1	72	80	4	125
B	176	85	0	8	16	0	310	188	186	2	1	14	0	0	125	92	20	87
C	122	60	0	63	50	0	293	115	306	0	4	35	1	1	58	75	4	122
D	70	28	0	248	94	0	234	66	231	1	19	26	0	37	74	64	6	111
E	59	23	0	375	118	0	142	85	277	3	7	45	0	9	33	31	1	102
F	85	39	0	260	105	0	235	89	222	4	11	26	0	9	67	42	2	113
G	57	21	1	294	92	0	173	80	281	0	8	25	0	10	115	43	5	105
H	114	26	0	229	84	0	215	107	245	0	10	39	0	22	64	38	2	114
I	75	30	3	250	94	0	254	71	214	0	18	36	1	46	91	30	2	95
J	50	27	0	323	102	0	179	100	251	1	21	33	0	22	44	21	5	91
K	70	26	1	247	99	0	245	84	261	1	18	28	1	34	60	34	3	97
L	54	28	1	337	107	0	246	92	195	2	23	23	0	27	40	21	2	111
M	100	60	0	103	69	0	234	105	312	3	1	36	0	6	53	57	6	165
O	81	53	0	182	100	0	188	92	329	4	4	48	0	4	50	32	7	136
P	91	55	0	134	77	0	207	118	306	1	12	37	0	0	50	64	7	151
Q	66	44	0	203	107	0	241	100	258	0	9	37	0	17	54	45	5	123
R	88	38	0	213	87	0	213	102	262	4	14	48	0	10	60	43	4	123
S	80	40	0	295	80	0	178	83	294	3	10	38	0	6	45	45	2	111

Actual (rows) / Predicted (columns)

FIGURE 5.26   Confusion matrix using LSTM on the WISDM dataset.

Confusion Matrix

Actual \ Predicted	A	B	C	D	E	F	G	H	I	J	K	L	M	O	P	Q	R	S
A	0.10	0.05	0.00	0.04	0.04	0.00	0.20	0.11	0.22	0.00	0.00	0.02	0.00	0.00	0.05	0.06	0.00	0.10
B	0.13	0.06	0.00	0.01	0.01	0.00	0.24	0.14	0.14	0.00	0.00	0.01	0.00	0.00	0.10	0.07	0.02	0.07
C	0.09	0.05	0.00	0.05	0.04	0.00	0.22	0.09	0.23	0.00	0.00	0.03	0.00	0.00	0.04	0.06	0.00	0.09
D	0.05	0.02	0.00	0.19	0.07	0.00	0.18	0.05	0.18	0.00	0.01	0.02	0.00	0.03	0.06	0.05	0.00	0.08
E	0.05	0.02	0.00	0.29	0.09	0.00	0.11	0.06	0.21	0.00	0.01	0.03	0.00	0.01	0.03	0.02	0.00	0.08
F	0.06	0.03	0.00	0.20	0.08	0.00	0.18	0.07	0.17	0.00	0.01	0.02	0.00	0.01	0.05	0.03	0.00	0.09
G	0.04	0.02	0.00	0.22	0.07	0.00	0.13	0.06	0.21	0.00	0.01	0.02	0.00	0.01	0.09	0.03	0.00	0.08
H	0.09	0.02	0.00	0.17	0.06	0.00	0.16	0.08	0.19	0.00	0.01	0.03	0.00	0.02	0.05	0.03	0.00	0.09
I	0.06	0.02	0.00	0.19	0.07	0.00	0.19	0.05	0.16	0.00	0.01	0.03	0.00	0.04	0.07	0.02	0.00	0.07
J	0.04	0.02	0.00	0.25	0.08	0.00	0.14	0.08	0.20	0.00	0.02	0.03	0.00	0.02	0.03	0.02	0.00	0.07
K	0.05	0.02	0.00	0.19	0.08	0.00	0.19	0.06	0.20	0.00	0.01	0.02	0.00	0.03	0.05	0.03	0.00	0.07
L	0.04	0.02	0.00	0.26	0.08	0.00	0.19	0.07	0.15	0.00	0.02	0.02	0.00	0.02	0.03	0.02	0.00	0.08
M	0.08	0.05	0.00	0.08	0.05	0.00	0.18	0.08	0.24	0.00	0.00	0.03	0.00	0.00	0.04	0.04	0.00	0.13
O	0.06	0.04	0.00	0.14	0.08	0.00	0.14	0.07	0.25	0.00	0.00	0.04	0.00	0.00	0.04	0.02	0.01	0.10
P	0.07	0.04	0.00	0.10	0.06	0.00	0.16	0.09	0.23	0.00	0.01	0.03	0.00	0.00	0.04	0.05	0.01	0.12
Q	0.05	0.03	0.00	0.16	0.08	0.00	0.18	0.08	0.20	0.00	0.01	0.03	0.00	0.01	0.04	0.03	0.00	0.09
R	0.07	0.03	0.00	0.16	0.07	0.00	0.16	0.08	0.20	0.00	0.01	0.04	0.00	0.01	0.05	0.03	0.00	0.09
S	0.06	0.03	0.00	0.23	0.06	0.00	0.14	0.06	0.22	0.00	0.01	0.03	0.00	0.00	0.03	0.03	0.00	0.08

FIGURE 5.27　Normalized confusion matrix using LSTM on the WISDM dataset.

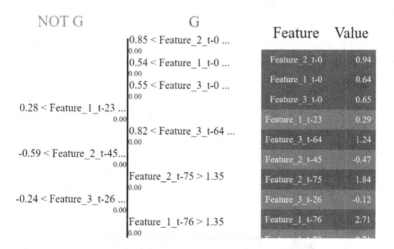

FIGURE 5.28　LIME explanation of a test sample using LSTM model on WISDM dataset.

5.1.5 Real-Time HAR Using Wearable Sensor

For real-time human activity recognition, MetaMotionR is used. The sensor is developed by MbientLab. The MetaMotionR sensor has compact design and a comprehensive suite of internal sensors, making it a good tool for various applications. The MetaMotionR sensor is equipped with a range of internal sensors, including accelerometers, gyroscopes, and magnetometers. These sensors collectively provide a wealth of data related to motion, orientation, and environmental conditions. The accelerometer measures acceleration forces, the gyroscope captures rotational rates, and the magnetometer detects magnetic fields. The combination of these sensors enables precise motion tracking and orientation sensing in three-dimensional space. One of the nice features of MetaMotionR is its ability to offer real-time data through wireless connectivity. The sensor supports Bluetooth Low Energy (BLE), facilitating seamless communication with other devices such as smartphones, tablets, or computers. This wireless capability is crucial for applications that require immediate access to data, enabling users to monitor and analyze sensor information remotely. Developers can access the data provided by MetaMotionR's internal sensors through MbientLab's software development kits (SDKs) and APIs (Application Programming Interfaces) such as https://mbientlab.com/tutorials/ and https://github.com/mbientlab/ MetaWear-SDK-Python. The GitHub repository is used in this work for real-time development of activity recognition.

These resources provide a set of tools and libraries that facilitate communication with the sensor, data acquisition, and the implementation of custom algorithms for processing and interpreting sensor data. The accelerometer data, for instance, can be utilized to measure changes in velocity and acceleration, making it valuable for applications such as activity tracking, gesture recognition, and impact detection. The gyroscope data enables the tracking of rotational movements, which is essential for applications involving orientation sensing, robotics, and virtual reality. The magnetometer data contributes to the sensor's ability to detect changes in magnetic fields, finding applications in compass functionality and orientation calibration. In healthcare, the sensor's data can be utilized for monitoring physical rehabilitation exercises. The precise motion tracking capabilities allow healthcare professionals to assess the quality and correctness of movements during rehabilitation, aiding in personalized treatment plans.

The MetaMotionR sensor's internal sensors, coupled with its wireless connectivity and developer-friendly resources, make it a valuable tool in a wide range of industries. Its compact form factor, rechargeable battery, and comprehensive documentation contribute to its accessibility for both seasoned developers and those new to sensor integration. Figure 5.29 shows the wearable sensor and how it was worn for real time human activity recognition. Figure 5.30 demonstrates the real time recognition results using the wearable sensor and machine learning where the RGB images are to show the ground truth only.

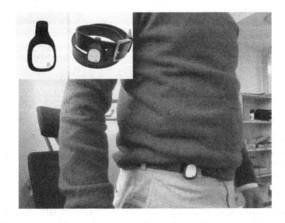

FIGURE 5.29 Wearable sensor and how it was worn for real time human activity recognition.

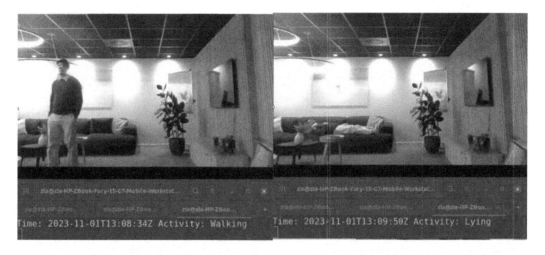

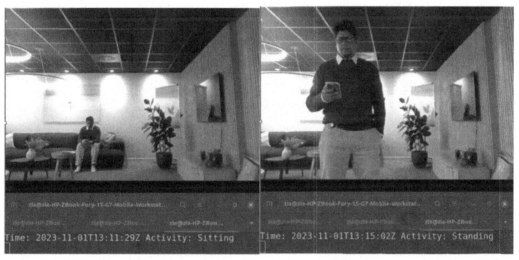

FIGURE 5.30   Real time human activity recognition using wearable sensor.

The data collection using the MbientLab sensor can be done as

```
# usage: python3 stream _ acc _ gyro _ bmi270.py
from __future__ import print_function
from mbientlab.metawear import MetaWear, libmetawear, parse_value
from mbientlab.metawear.cbindings import *
from time import sleep
from threading import Event

import platform
import sys
import re
import pandas as pd

if sys.version _ info[0] == 2:
    range = xrange
```

```
AX = []
AY = []
AZ = []
GX = []
GY = []
GZ= []


class State:
    # init
    def __init__(self, device):
        self.device = device
        self.samples = 0
        self.accCallback = FnVoid_VoidP_DataP(self.acc_data_handler)
        self.gyroCallback = FnVoid_VoidP_DataP(self.gyro_data_handler)


    # acc callback
    def acc_data_handler(self, ctx, data):
        #print("ACC: %s -> %s" % (self.device.address,
parse_value(data)))
        self.samples+= 1
        s = str(parse_value(data))
        values =re.findall("\d+\.\d+",s)
        parsed_val = ([float(x) for x in values])
        AX.append(parsed_val[0])
        AY.append(parsed_val[1])
        AZ.append(parsed_val[2])

    # gyro callback
    def gyro_data_handler(self, ctx, data):
        #print("GYRO: %s -> %s" % (self.device.address,
parse_value(data)))
        self.samples+= 1
        s = str(parse_value(data))
        values =re.findall("\d+\.\d+",s)
        parsed_val = ([float(x) for x in values])
        GX.append(parsed_val[0])
        GY.append(parsed_val[1])
        GZ.append(parsed_val[2])


states = []

# connect
for i in range(len(sys.argv) - 1):
    d = MetaWear(sys.argv[i + 1])
    d.connect()
    print("Connected to " + d.address + " over " + ("USB" if
d.usb.is_connected else "BLE"))
    states.append(State(d))

# configure
for s in states:
```

```
    print("Configuring device")
    libmetawear.mbl_mw_settings_set_connection_parameters(s.
device.board, 7.5, 7.5, 0, 6000)
    sleep(1.5)

    # setup acc
    #libmetawear.mbl_mw_acc_set_odr(s.device.board, 50.0) #
Generic call
    libmetawear.mbl_mw_acc_bmi270_set_odr(s.device.board,
AccBmi270Odr._50Hz) # BMI 270 specific call
    libmetawear.mbl_mw_acc_bosch_set_range(s.device.board,
AccBoschRange._4G)
    libmetawear.mbl_mw_acc_write_acceleration_config(s.device.board)

    # setup gyro
    libmetawear.mbl_mw_gyro_bmi270_set_range(s.device.board,
GyroBoschRange._1000dps);
    libmetawear.mbl_mw_gyro_bmi270_set_odr(s.device.board,
GyroBoschOdr._50Hz);
    libmetawear.mbl_mw_gyro_bmi270_write_config(s.device.board);

    # get acc and subscribe
    acc = libmetawear.mbl_mw_acc_get_acceleration_data_signal(s.
device.board)
    libmetawear.mbl_mw_datasignal_subscribe(acc, None,
s.accCallback)

    # get gyro and subscribe
    gyro = libmetawear.mbl_mw_gyro_bmi270_get_rotation_data_
signal(s.device.board)
    libmetawear.mbl_mw_datasignal_subscribe(gyro, None,
s.gyroCallback)

    # start acc
    libmetawear.mbl_mw_acc_enable_acceleration_sampling(s.device.
board)

    libmetawear.mbl_mw_acc_start(s.device.board)
    # start gyro
    libmetawear.mbl_mw_gyro_bmi270_enable_rotation_sampling(s.
device.board)
    libmetawear.mbl_mw_gyro_bmi270_start(s.device.board)

# sleep
sleep(30.0)

# stop
for s in states:
    libmetawear.mbl_mw_acc_stop(s.device.board)
    libmetawear.mbl_mw_acc_disable_acceleration_sampling(s.device.
board)
```

```
    libmetawear.mbl _ mw _ gyro _ bmi270 _ stop(s.device.board)
    libmetawear.mbl_mw_gyro_bmi270_disable_rotation_sampling
(s.device.board)

    acc = libmetawear.mbl _ mw _ acc _ get _ acceleration _ data _
signal(s.device.board)
    libmetawear.mbl_mw_datasignal_unsubscribe(acc)

    gyro = libmetawear.mbl _ mw _ gyro _ bmi270 _ get _ rotation _
data _ signal(s.device.board)
    libmetawear.mbl_mw_datasignal_unsubscribe(gyro)

    libmetawear.mbl _ mw _ debug _ disconnect(s.device.board)

# recap
print("Total Samples Received")
for s in states:
    #print("%s -> %d" % (s.device.address, s.samples))
    L = min(len(AX), len(GX))
    data = {'AX':AX[0:L], 'AY':AY[0:L], 'AZ':AZ[0:L],
'GX':GX[0:L], 'GY':GY[0:L], 'GZ':GZ[0:L]}
    df = pd.DataFrame(data)
    #print(L)
    #print(df.head())

    df.to_csv('Standing.csv', mode='a', index=False, header=False)
```

Training the model can be done as follows:

```
import pandas as pd
import tensorflow as tf
import numpy as np
import math

#Process Standing Data
df = pd.read_csv('Standing.csv')
Data1 = df.to_numpy()
S = math.floor(Data1.shape[0]/300)
L = S*300
D = Data1[0:L,:]
D1 = np.reshape(D, (S,300,6))
Y1 = np.zeros((D1.shape[0], 4))
Y1[:,0]=1

#Process Sitting Data
df = pd.read_csv('Sitting.csv')
Data2 = df.to_numpy()
S = math.floor(Data2.shape[0]/300)
L = S*300
D = Data2[0:L,:]
```

```
D2 = np.reshape(D, (S,300,6))
Y2 = np.zeros((D2.shape[0], 4))
Y2[:,1]=1

#Process Lying Data
df = pd.read_csv('Lying.csv')
Data3 = df.to_numpy()
S = math.floor(Data3.shape[0]/300)
L = S*300
D = Data3[0:L,:]
D3 = np.reshape(D, (S,300,6))
Y3 = np.zeros((D3.shape[0], 4))
Y3[:,2]=1

#Process Walking Data
df = pd.read_csv('Walking.csv')
Data4 = df.to_numpy()
S = math.floor(Data4.shape[0]/300)
L = S*300
D = Data4[0:L,:]
D4 = np.reshape(D, (S,300,6))
Y4 = np.zeros((D4.shape[0], 4))
Y4[:,3]=1

X = np.concatenate((D1, D2, D3, D4), axis=0)
Y = np.concatenate((Y1, Y2, Y3, Y4), axis=0)

from sklearn.model_selection import train_test_split

trainx, testx, trainy, testy = train_test_split(X, Y, test_
size=0.20, random_state=42)

model = tf.keras.Sequential([
        tf.keras.Input((300, 6)),
        tf.keras.layers.LSTM(20),
        tf.keras.layers.Dense(4, activation = 'softmax')
        ])

model.compile(loss = 'categorical_crossentropy',
                optimizer = 'rmsprop',
                metrics = ['accuracy'])
model.summary()

model.fit(trainx, trainy, batch_size=20, epochs=100)

y_pred=model.predict(testx)
y_pred_classes = np.argmax(y_pred, axis=1)

y_true = np.argmax(testy, axis=1)
```

```
from sklearn.metrics import confusion_matrix
conf=confusion_matrix(y_true, y_pred_classes)

model.save_weights("HAR.h5")

data_columns = [ 'Feature_{}'.format(x) for x in range(1,7)]
from lime import lime_tabular

explainer = lime_tabular.RecurrentTabularExplainer(trainx,
training_labels=trainy, feature_names=data_columns,
                            discretize_continuous=True,
                            class_names=['Standing',
'Sitting', 'Lying', 'Walking'], discretizer='decile')

exp = explainer.explain_instance(testx[20], model.predict, num_
features=6, labels=(1,))
exp.show_in_notebook()
```

After generating the model, the real-time activity recognition can be done as

```
# usage: python3 stream_acc_gyro_bmi270.py [mac1] [mac2] … [mac(n)]
from __future__ import print_function
from mbientlab.metawear import MetaWear, libmetawear, parse_value
from mbientlab.metawear.cbindings import *
import os
os.system("clear")
from time import sleep
from threading import Event
import platform
import sys
import re
import pandas as pd
import tensorflow as tf
import numpy as np
import math
import os
import time
import datetime
from datetime import timedelta
import os
import pytz

os.environ['TZ'] = 'Norway/Oslo'
time.tzset()

AX = []
AY = []
AZ = []
GX = []
GY = []
GZ = []
```

```python
class State:
    # init
    def __init__(self, device):
        self.device = device
        self.samples = 0
        self.accCallback = FnVoid_VoidP_DataP(self.acc_data_
handler)
        self.gyroCallback = FnVoid_VoidP_DataP(self.
gyro_data_handler)

    # acc callback
    def acc_data_handler(self, ctx, data):
        #print("ACC: %s -> %s" % (self.device.address,
parse_value(data)))
        self.samples+= 1
        s = str(parse_value(data))
        values =re.findall("\d+\.\d+",s)
        parsed_val = ([float(x) for x in values])
        AX.append(parsed_val[0])
        AY.append(parsed_val[1])
        AZ.append(parsed_val[2])

    # gyro callback
    def gyro_data_handler(self, ctx, data):
        #print("GYRO: %s -> %s" % (self.device.address,
parse_value(data)))
        self.samples+= 1
        s = str(parse_value(data))
        values =re.findall("\d+\.\d+",s)
        parsed_val = ([float(x) for x in values])
        GX.append(parsed_val[0])
        GY.append(parsed_val[1])
        GZ.append(parsed_val[2])
states = []
os.system("clear")
# connect
for i in range(len(sys.argv) - 1):
    d = MetaWear(sys.argv[i + 1])
    d.connect()
    print("Connected to " + d.address + " over " + ("USB" if
d.usb.is_connected else "BLE"))
    states.append(State(d))
os.system("clear")
# configure
for s in states:
    print("Configuring device")
    libmetawear.mbl_mw_settings_set_connection_parameters(s.
device.board, 7.5, 7.5, 0, 6000)
    sleep(1.5)
```

```
    # setup acc
    #libmetawear.mbl_mw_acc_set_odr(s.device.board, 50.0) #
Generic call
    libmetawear.mbl_mw_acc_bmi270_set_odr(s.device.board,
AccBmi270Odr._50Hz) # BMI 270 specific call
    libmetawear.mbl_mw_acc_bosch_set_range(s.device.board,
AccBoschRange._4G)
    libmetawear.mbl_mw_acc_write_acceleration_config(s.device.
board)

    # setup gyro
    libmetawear.mbl_mw_gyro_bmi270_set_range(s.device.board,
GyroBoschRange._1000dps);
    libmetawear.mbl_mw_gyro_bmi270_set_odr(s.device.board,
GyroBoschOdr._50Hz);
    libmetawear.mbl_mw_gyro_bmi270_write_config(s.device.board);

    # get acc and subscribe
    acc = libmetawear.mbl_mw_acc_get_acceleration_data_signal(s.
device.board)
    libmetawear.mbl_mw_datasignal_subscribe(acc, None,
s.accCallback)

    # get gyro and subscribe
    gyro = libmetawear.mbl_mw_gyro_bmi270_get_rotation_data_
signal(s.device.board)
    libmetawear.mbl_mw_datasignal_subscribe(gyro, None,
s.gyroCallback)

    # start acc
    libmetawear.mbl_mw_acc_enable_acceleration_sampling(s.device.
board)
    libmetawear.mbl_mw_acc_start(s.device.board)

    # start gyro
    libmetawear.mbl_mw_gyro_bmi270_enable_rotation_sampling(s.
device.board)
    libmetawear.mbl_mw_gyro_bmi270_start(s.device.board)

# sleep
sleep(10.0)
os.system("clear")
# stop
for s in states:
    libmetawear.mbl_mw_acc_stop(s.device.board)
    libmetawear.mbl_mw_acc_disable_acceleration_sampling(s.device.
board)

    libmetawear.mbl_mw_gyro_bmi270_stop(s.device.board)
```

```
    libmetawear.mbl_mw_gyro_bmi270_disable_rotation_sampling
(s.device.board)

    acc = libmetawear.mbl_mw_acc_get_acceleration_data_
signal(s.device.board)
    libmetawear.mbl_mw_datasignal_unsubscribe(acc)

    gyro = libmetawear.mbl_mw_gyro_bmi270_get_rotation_
data_signal(s.device.board)
    libmetawear.mbl_mw_datasignal_unsubscribe(gyro)

    libmetawear.mbl_mw_debug_disconnect(s.device.board)

# recap
#print("Total Samples Received")
for s in states:
    L = min(len(AX), len(GX))
    data = {'AX':AX[0:L], 'AY':AY[0:L], 'AZ':AZ[0:L],
'GX':GX[0:L], 'GY':GY[0:L], 'GZ':GZ[0:L]}
    df = pd.DataFrame(data)
    Data1 = df.to_numpy()
    S = math.floor(Data1.shape[0]/300)
    L = S*300
    D = Data1[0:L,:]
    D1 = np.reshape(D, (S,300,6))
    model = tf.keras.Sequential([
        tf.keras.Input((300, 6)),
        tf.keras.layers.LSTM(20),
        tf.keras.layers.Dense(4, activation = 'softmax')
        ])
    model.compile(loss = 'categorical_crossentropy',
                optimizer = 'rmsprop',
                metrics = ['accuracy'])
    model.load_weights("HAR.h5")
    y_pred=model.predict(D1)
    y_pred_classes = np.argmax(y_pred, axis=1)
    #print(y_pred_classes)
    os.system("clear")
    act=y_pred_classes[0]
    now = datetime.datetime.now(pytz.timezone('Europe/Oslo'))
    Good_time= now.strftime('%Y-%m-%dT%H:%M:%SZ')
    if (act==0):
        print("Time: "+Good_time+ " Activity: " + "Standing")
    if (act==1):
        print("Time: "+Good_time+ " Activity: " + "Sitting")
    if (act==2):
        print("Time: "+Good_time+ " Activity: " +"Lying")
    if (act==3):
        print("Time: "+Good_time+ " Activity: " +"Walking")
```

5.2 VIDEO CAMERA-BASED BEHAVIOR RECOGNITION

Video data serves as the predominant ambient sensor technology in assisted living for monitoring and analyzing diverse human activities [27–36]. Alongside facilitating the development of crucial applications, video recognition allows for the detection of various human activities. In public spaces such as airports and subway stations, automated surveillance systems must identify abnormal and suspicious behavior in addition to normal activities. For instance, offering real-time monitoring for patients, children, and the elderly, video-based behavior recognition aids in identifying potential issues. The development of human–computer interfaces and vision-based intelligent systems has presented significant challenges. Tracking and understanding a person's behavior through video recordings from multiple cameras is a critical and complex problem. Vision-based behavior recognition finds applications in human–computer interaction, user interface design, robot learning, and surveillance, among others. Substantial global research employs different camera types, including RGB, stereo, infrared, and multiple cameras, to explore various methods for vision-based activity recognition. The computational process in vision-based activity recognition typically involves four steps: detection, tracking, recognition, and evaluation of human activity.

Considering the human body's composition of interconnected limbs and joints, acquiring 3-D joint angle information yields considerably more robust features than conventional binary silhouette features, leading to a notable enhancement in human body activity recognition. To overcome the limitations of binary and depth silhouettes, utilizing joint-angle information from a 3-D whole body model proves to be a more effective method for identifying human activity. The conventional approach involves a predefined environment with optical markers on a subject, enabling the capture of 3-D human body configuration by multiple cameras. Inverse kinematic analysis extrapolates body joint angles from the three-dimensional coordinates of the markers. However, this marker-based system is restrictive and unsuitable for daily activity monitoring. To address this limitation, this study proposes a marker-free Human Activity Recognition (HAR) system. There has been increasing focus on capturing a 3-D configuration of the human body from images without markers. However, deploying multiple cameras at various angles simultaneously and synchronizing them poses challenges. This approach is less practical for everyday use. Consequently, single-camera-based body skeleton tracking is gaining popularity day by day.

OpenPose emerged from the Carnegie Mellon Perceptual Computing Lab's research, a group dedicated to advancing technologies related to human perception and interaction. The goal of the project was to create a resilient and adaptable algorithm proficient in accurately detecting and tracking human body movements from images or video frames. The development of OpenPose involved harnessing deep neural networks, computational models inspired by the structure and function of the human brain. These networks underwent training on extensive datasets containing diverse human poses and movements. This training facilitated OpenPose in learning complex patterns and relationships within the human skeletal structure, enabling it to generalize and accurately estimate poses in real-world scenarios. The algorithm's structure is designed to recognize crucial joints and body parts, such as arms, legs, and torso, in both 2D and 3D space. This comprehensive comprehension of the human body's spatial configuration contributes to the algorithm's exceptional accuracy in pose estimation.

Researchers and developers behind OpenPose continually refined and optimized the algorithm through iterative testing and feedback loops. They addressed challenges associated with varied body types, clothing variations, and environmental conditions to enhance the algorithm's robustness and applicability across different contexts. OpenPose's development also benefited from collaborations and contributions from the broader research community. The open-source nature of the project permitted researchers, developers, and enthusiasts globally to contribute to its enhancement, resulting in a collective effort to advance the capabilities of the algorithm. The collaborative and open-source nature of the project has played a pivotal role in its evolution and widespread adoption in diverse fields.

It is excellent at understanding how people move in pictures and videos by looking at critical joints and body parts with impressive accuracy. Beyond just showing poses, OpenPose excels in understanding human behavior. It acts like a detective, paying attention to every detail of a person's moves. This versatility allows it to be applied in various fields. In healthcare, OpenPose monitors patients during physical therapy exercises, ensuring they perform them correctly by tracking their movements. In surveillance, OpenPose analyzes video footage to spot unusual movements or gestures that could indicate a security concern, enhancing public safety in places like airports. For human–computer interaction, OpenPose interprets how users move or gesture, making technology more user-friendly. For example, you could control a presentation by waving your hand. OpenPose helps teachers understand how engaged students are during a lesson by tracking their body language. In entertainment and gaming, OpenPose adds excitement by capturing real-world movements. Imagine playing a video game where your character mimics your gestures, making gaming more immersive.

Overall, OpenPose is more than just a tech tool; it's a gateway to a world of possibilities. Its ability to understand and recognize human behavior opens up new avenues across different fields, making our interactions with technology more natural and exciting. As technology advances, OpenPose stands at the forefront, promising a future where our devices understand us through what we say or type and how we move and express ourselves. It's an exciting step towards a more interactive relationship between humans and technology.

Figures 5.31 and 5.32 show the real-time skeleton tracking from RGB and thermal cameras. One important thing to note is that it works even in the dark, whereas RGB or depth cameras don't. Hence, it can be applied 24 hours observation of people such as elderly to avoid unexpected event such as fall in any time.

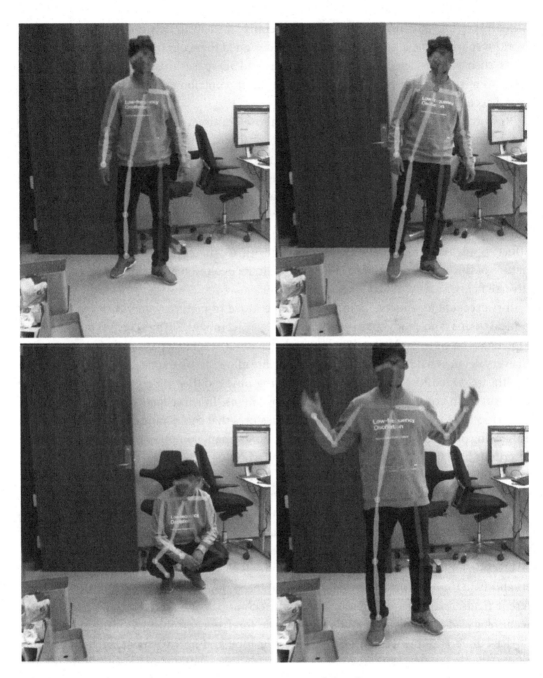

FIGURE 5.31   Real-time pose estimation using RGB camera and OpenPose.

5.3 AMBIENT SENSOR-BASED BEHAVIOR RECOGNITION

A smart home provides independence and comfort to the residents by using all technological devices interconnected within the network, capable of communicating and learning through the user's habits, providing an interactive environment for the residents [37]–[62]. Based on the widely used Benchmarks of the Center for Advanced Studies in Adaptive Systems (CASAS), the reliability of the proposed approach for activity recognition is examined in a smart home scenario. The CASAS datasets are widely used and investigated by

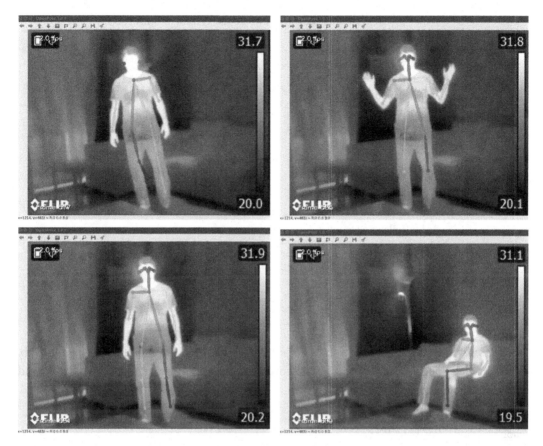

FIGURE 5.32   Real time pose estimation using thermal camera and OpenPose during dark.

researchers using supervised algorithms; however, there is still a lack of studies examining the use of deep learning approaches which incorporate temporal information into deep learning approaches. Washington State University introduced the CASAS datasets [61], and the testbed bright apartment used in the CASAS smart home project consisted of three apartments with three bedrooms, one bathroom, a kitchen, and a living/dining area. Sensors (such as motion, temperature, and door sensors) and actuators were installed in each apartment to monitor and report on the surrounding environment. Among all available CASAS datasets, Milan is selected to show, but others can also be used. The Milan dataset contains sensor data collected in the home of a volunteer adult. The residents were a woman and a dog. The woman's children visited on several occasions. Sensor events were generated from motion (M), door closure (D), and temperature (T) sensors.

As part of the preprocessing process of the dataset, filters were performed from the CASAS datasets. The input features included raw data from various smart home sensors (e.g., M, D, T). The data aggregate was performed to encapsulate all changes in sensor status considering the lapse in time between the beginning and end of the human activity. This processing results in an input matrix of sensor events associated with each activity, which will be used as features in the subsequent machine learning process. The input data was used to develop a class-membership prediction model based on the LSTM. Table 5.5 shows different events from the Milan site of the dataset.

TABLE 5.5   CASAS Dataset Events with Residents from the Milan Site

Milan:
Chores: Work
Desk Activity: Work
Morning Meds: Take medicine
Eve Meds: Take medicine
Sleep: Sleep
Read Relax
Watch TV: Relax
Leave Home Leave Home
Dining Rm Activity: Eat
Kitchen Activity: Cook
Bed to Toilet: Bed to toilet
Master Bathroom: Bathing
Guest Bathroom: Bathing
Master Bedroom
Activity: Other
Meditate: Other

The following modified code is developed based on the Github code at https://github.com/danielelic/deep-casas/tree/master, for milan dataset but other dataset can also be used exploring the repository.

```
import argparse
import tensorflow.keras
import numpy as np
from sklearn.metrics import confusion_matrix,
classification_report
from sklearn.model_selection import KFold
from tensorflow.keras import layers
from tensorflow.keras.models import Sequential, load_model
from tensorflow.keras.layers import Embedding
from tensorflow.keras.layers import Dense, LSTM, Bidirectional
from sklearn.model_selection import train_test_split

import data

data_dim = 2000
timesteps =1
num_classes = 10

# expected input data shape: (batch_size, timesteps, data_dim)
model = Sequential()
model.add(LSTM(50, return_sequences=True,
            input_shape=(timesteps, data_dim)))  # returns a
sequence of vectors of dimension 32
model.add(LSTM(50, return_sequences=True))  # returns a sequence
of vectors of dimension 32
model.add(LSTM(50, return_sequences=True))  # returns a sequence
of vectors of dimension 32
```

```
model.add(LSTM(50))   # return a single vector of dimension 32
model.add(Dense(num_classes, activation='softmax'))

model.compile(loss='categorical_crossentropy',
              optimizer='rmsprop',
              metrics=['accuracy'])

data_x, data_y, dictActivities = data.getData('milan')
#for cairo
#data_x, data_y, dictActivities = data.getData('cairo')

from tensorflow.keras.utils import to_categorical
data_y = to_categorical(data_y, dtype ="uint8")

X_train, X_test, Y_train, Y_test = train_test_split(data_x,
data_y, test_size=0.3)
X_train, X_val, Y_train, Y_val = train_test_split(X_train, Y_
train, test_size=0.1)

x_train=np.reshape(X_train, (X_train.shape[0], timesteps,
data_dim))
x_test=np.reshape(X_test, (X_test.shape[0], timesteps, data_dim))
y_train=Y_train
y_test=Y_test
x_val=np.reshape(X_val, (X_val.shape[0], timesteps, data_dim))
y_val=Y_val
#model.summary()
model.fit(x_train, y_train, validation_data=(x_val, y_val),
epochs=500, batch_size=100)

score, acc = model.evaluate(x_test, y_test,
                            batch_size=100)
print('Test score:', score)
print('Test accuracy:', acc)

import numpy as np
from lime import lime_tabular
data_columns = [ 'Feature_{}'.format(x) for x in range(1,2001)]

explainer = lime_tabular.RecurrentTabularExplainer(x_train,
training_labels=y_train, feature_names=data_columns,
                                                   discretize_
continuous=True,
                                                   class_
names=['A1', 'A2','A3', 'A4','A5', 'A6', 'A7', 'A8', 'A9', 'A10'],

discretizer='decile')
exp = explainer.explain_instance(x_test[350], model.predict, num_
features=100, labels=(0,))
exp.show_in_notebook()
```

The output is *Test accuracy: 0.45*. Lime generates the following explanation SHOWN IN Figure 5.33 where it shows that the activity is A1 which is work.

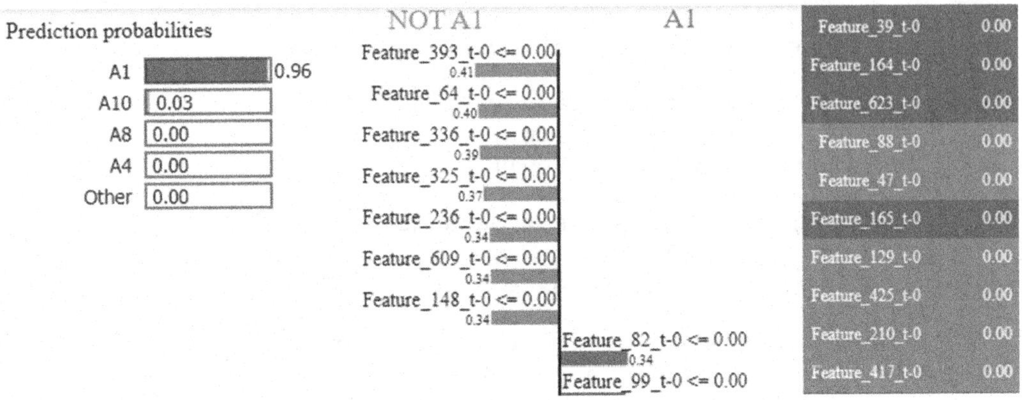

FIGURE 5.33   LIME explanation using LSTM on the Milan site of CASAS dataset.

5.3.1 Real-Time Home Monitoring Using Ambient Sensors

In the world of smart homes, ambient sensors step into the spotlight, bringing a multitude of practical applications that go beyond just convenience—they make our homes safer, more energy-efficient, and smarter. These devices, designed to pick up changes in our surroundings, have become vital players in the modern design and functionality of smart homes. Motion sensors, for instance, are like vigilant watchers, spotting any movement in and around our homes and prompting security measures like alarms or notifications. Paired with smart surveillance systems, these sensors provide real-time updates, letting us keep an eye on our homes even when we're away. Our well-being also gets a boost from ambient sensors, especially air quality sensors. These diligent monitors keep tabs on our indoor air, flagging any pollutants or allergens. By alerting us to poor air quality, these sensors give us the power to act—adjusting ventilation or purifying the air. Water management becomes a breeze with ambient sensors in the mix. Leak detection sensors, for instance, can sense water leaks and give us a heads up before things get messy. Sound sensors pick up on unusual noises, triggering responses like turning on lights or sending alerts. Ambient sensors in smart home monitoring make our homes more functional, efficient, and safe. From keeping our homes at the perfect temperature to optimizing lighting, ensuring security, and monitoring our health, these sensors are the backbone of a more intelligent and responsive living environment. As technology marches forward, we can expect ambient sensors to continue evolving, offering even more sophisticated solutions for those who seek comfort, convenience, and sustainability in their homes.

As an experiment, ambient sensors and gateway are used [63]. White-label sensors and gateways, like those offered by [63], allow businesses to brand and customize these devices as their own. These products serve as a foundation for companies looking to enter the Internet of Things (IoT) market without the burden of developing their hardware from scratch. White-label sensors can seamlessly integrate into diverse applications, allowing businesses to collect valuable data on environmental conditions, occupancy, or other relevant parameters. The gateway is a central command center, enabling efficient communication between sensors and the broader IoT network. Figure 5.34 shows a sample dashboard of a gateway and the sensor devices [63]. Figure 5.35 shows how the sensors and gateway

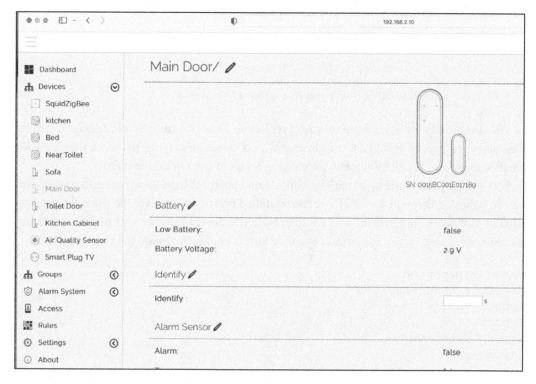

FIGURE 5.34   Innovative white label sensors gateway dashboard of a sample smart home gateway.

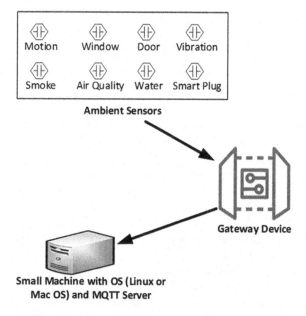

FIGURE 5.35   Combined different sensors and devices for a sample smart home sensor setup.

2023-12-22T15:06:17Z Vibration Sofa/Bed False

2023-12-22T15:06:19Z Main Door Opening True

2023-12-22T15:06:22Z Main Door Opening False

FIGURE 5.36   Example real-time output from a sample smart home setup.

can be combined with a machine to collect real-time data with the help of Message Queuing Telemetry Transport (MQTT), a lightweight and open messaging protocol designed for small sensors and mobile devices with varying levels of network connectivity.

Following Python code on a small machine shows how real-time data from different devices can be collected through an MQTT server installed on the small machine since the gateway used in this work supports an MQTT interface. The device number can be initially determined empirically. Figure 5.36 shows example outputs using the following code structure.

```
#!/usr/bin/python
import subprocess, sys
import yaml
import time
import datetime
import pytz

#cmd is mosquito command to get the device info from the server.
 p = subprocess.Popen(cmd, shell=True, stdout=subprocess.
PIPE,universal_newlines=True)

power=0
Temp=[]
Tm =0
Humid=[]
Hm =0

while True:
    try:
        T = p.stdout.readline()
        T = T.strip()
        x =  str(bytes(T, encoding="utf-8"))
#       dev = "Find the device number from x by parsing the string"

        if(dev=='1' and (name == 'Occupancy') and  (value=='True' or
value=='False')):
            Sensor = "Kicten Area"

        if(dev=='2' and (name == 'Occupancy') and  (value=='True' or
value=='False')):
            Sensor = "Bed Area"

        if(dev=='3' and (name == 'Occupancy') and  (value=='True' or
value=='False')):
```

```
        Sensor = "Toilet Area"

    if(dev=='4' and (value=='True' or value=='False') and name ==
'Vibration Alarm'):
        Sensor = "Vibration Sofa/Bed"

    if(dev=='5'and  (value=='True' or value=='False') and name ==
'Alarm'):
        Sensor = "Main Door Opening"

    if(dev=='6'and  (value=='True' or value=='False') and name ==
'Alarm'):
        Sensor = "Toilet Door Opening"

    if(dev=='7'and  (value=='True' or value=='False') and name ==
'Alarm'):
        Sensor = "Kitchen Cabinet Door Opening"

    if(dev=='8' and (name == 'Relative Humidity' or name == 'Air
quality - Level' or name == 'Air quality - Recommendation' or  name
== 'Measured Temperature')):
        Sensor = "Air Quality"

    if(dev=='9' and name == 'Instantaneous Energy Use'):
        Sensor = "SmartPlug"
#show time, sensor name and value of the senor
   now = datetime.datetime.now()
    print(now.strftime('%Y-%m-%dT%H:%M:%SZ') + " " + Sensor +
" " + value)
   except Exception:
      continue
```

5.3.2 Occupancy Prediction Dataset

The UCI Occupancy Detection dataset, found on the UCI Machine Learning Repository, is like a treasure chest for understanding when a room is occupied based on different environmental factors. With a hefty 20,560 instances collected over about a month, this dataset gives us a detailed look at how room occupancy is affected by different factors. In terms of the environment, the dataset considers basic matters such as temperature, humidity, light, and CO_2 levels. Temperature readings tell us about the room's warmth, humidity levels show how moist the air is, light readings give insights into how bright the room is, and CO_2 levels tell us about the air quality. A big deal in this dataset is whether or not a room is occupied. Each entry has a time stamp, telling us if the office room was in use or empty at that specific time. This binary way of labeling if a room is occupied or not makes the dataset great for teaching computer models to figure out if a room is being used or not.

The researchers can use this dataset to explore and create models. Their goal can be to figure out how changes in the environment affect whether a room is occupied. They might use machine learning models like Decision Trees, Support Vector Machines, or Deep

Neural Networks to predict if a room is occupied based on the recorded features. The dataset also considers time, letting researchers see how room occupancy changes over different times of the day, weekdays, or weekends. This time aspect is crucial for understanding when and how often a room gets used. It's like a puzzle piece for making smart buildings that know when to turn on lights, air conditioning, or heating to save energy.

The UCI Occupancy Detection dataset is like a guide for understanding when and why people are in a room. It helps make buildings smarter by using this information to save energy and keep things safe. Different visualization and machine learning algorithms can be coded as follows.

```python
import numpy as np
import pandas as pd
import seaborn as sns
import matplotlib.pyplot as plt
from sklearn.preprocessing import MinMaxScaler
from sklearn.metrics import accuracy_score, confusion_matrix,

# Load Dataset
datatest = pd.read_csv("./datatest.txt")
datatest2 = pd.read_csv("./datatest2.txt")
datatrain = pd.read_csv("./datatraining.txt")

# Normalize the input data

from sklearn.preprocessing import MinMaxScaler
scaler = MinMaxScaler()
columns = ['Temperature', 'Humidity', 'Light', 'CO2',
'HumidityRatio']
scaler.fit(np.array(datatrain[columns]))
datatest[columns] = scaler.transform(np.array(datatest[columns]))
datatest2[columns] = scaler.transform(np.
array(datatest2[columns]))
datatrain[columns] = scaler.transform(np.array(datatrain[columns]))

# Draw the box plot of the input data
plt.figure(figsize=(10,10))
ax = sns.boxplot(data=datatrain.drop(['date',
'Occupancy'],axis=1), orient="v", palette="Set1")

# Show the data correlation
corr = datatrain.corr()
plt.figure(figsize = (8,6))
sns.heatmap(corr, annot = True, cmap = 'crest', annot_kws={"size":
12})

# Show the Occupancy Distribution

sns.set(style="whitegrid")
```

```
plt.title("Occupancy Distribution", fontdict={'fontsize':14})
ax = sns.countplot(x="Occupancy", data=datatrain)

# Our data is unbalanced, so we need to find another relations
between features to strengthen our predictions. I have a question at
this point, is there any relation between occupancy and the hour of
the day? Let's look into it.

# Separate input and output columns
X_train = datatrain.drop(columns=['date', 'Occupancy'], axis=1)
y_train = datatrain['Occupancy']
X_validation = datatest.drop(columns=['date', 'Occupancy'],
axis=1)
y_validation = datatest['Occupancy']
X_test = datatest2.drop(columns=['date', 'Occupancy'], axis=1)
y_test = datatest2['Occupancy']

# Define a function to show confusion matrix and accuracy
def plot_confusion_matrix(y_test, y_preds):
    cm = confusion_matrix(y_test, y_preds)
    classes = ['No Occupancy', 'Occupancy']
    ax = sns.heatmap(cm, cbar=False, cmap="Blues", annot=True,
annot_kws={"size": 18}, fmt='g', xticklabels=classes,
yticklabels=classes)
    print(accuracy_score(y_test, y_preds))

#Apply KNN

from sklearn.neighbors import KNeighborsClassifier
knn = KNeighborsClassifier(n_neighbors = 5, metric = 'minkowski',
p = 2)
knn.fit(X_train, y_train)
y_preds = knn.predict(X_test)
plot_confusion_matrix(y_test, y_preds)

#Apply SVM

from sklearn.svm import SVC
svm_model = SVC()
svm_model.fit(X_train, y_train)
y_preds = svm_model.predict(X_test)
plot_confusion_matrix(y_test, y_preds)

#Apply Logistic Regression

from sklearn.linear _ model import LogisticRegression
logistic = LogisticRegression(random_state = 1, max_iter=10000)
logistic.fit(X_train, y_train)
y_preds = logistic.predict(X_test)
plot_confusion_matrix(y_test, y_preds)
```

```
#Apply AdaBoost

from sklearn.ensemble import AdaBoostClassifier
ada_boost = AdaBoostClassifier(n_estimators = 500, learning_rate =
0.02, random_state = 0)
ada_boost.fit(X_train, y_train)
y_preds = ada_boost.predict(X_test)
plot_confusion_matrix(y_test, y_preds)

# Apply LSTM

from tensorflow.keras.models import Sequential
from tensorflow.keras.layers import Dense
from tensorflow.keras.layers import LSTM
from tensorflow.keras.preprocessing import sequence

L =X _ train.shape
M = X_validation.shape
N = X_test.shape

X _ train = np.asarray(X _ train)
X_validation = np.asarray(X_validation)
X_test = np.asarray(X_test)

X _ train =X _ train.reshape(L[0], 1, L[1])
X_validation =X_validation.reshape(M[0], 1, M[1])
X_test =X_test.reshape(N[0], 1, N[1])

# create and fit the LSTM network
model = Sequential()
model.add(LSTM(10, input_shape=(1,5)))
model.add(Dense(1, activation='sigmoid'))
model.compile(optimizer='rmsprop',
              loss='binary_crossentropy',
              metrics=['accuracy'])
history = model.fit(X_train, y_train, epochs=200, batch_size=100,
verbose = 0)

y _ preds = model.predict(X _ test)
threshold = 0.5
y_preds = [1 if i >= threshold else 0 for i in y_preds]

plot _ confusion _ matrix(y _ test, y _ preds)

#Show model loss vs epochs
plt.plot(history.history['loss'], label='train_loss')
plt.title('Training  Loss')
plt.xlabel('Epoch')
plt.ylabel('Loss')
plt.legend()
plt.show()
```

Figures 5.37–5.40, and Table 5.6 reflects the outputs obtained using the above code. An overall observation in this case is, shallow machine learning overpowers LSTM by obtaining higher accuracy.

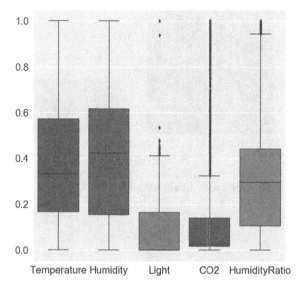

FIGURE 5.37   Box plot of the features in Occupancy dataset.

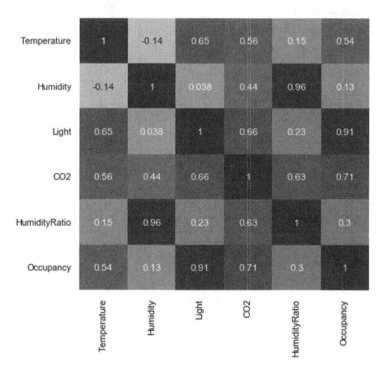

FIGURE 5.38   Correlation of Occupancy dataset using seaborn library.

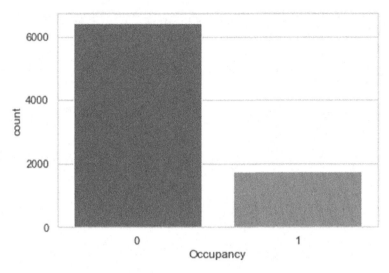

FIGURE 5.39 Distribution of samples with occupancy value 0 and 1.

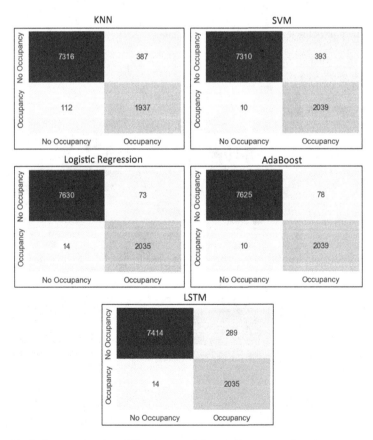

FIGURE 5.40 Confusion matrix using different approaches on Occupancy dataset.

TABLE 5.6 Accuracies of Different Machine Learning Approaches Codes on Occupancy Dataset

Approach	Accuracy
KNN	0.95
SVM	0.95
Logistic Regression	0.99
AdaBoost	0.99
LSTM	0.97

5.4 HEALTH STATUS MONITORING

The healthcare landscape has seen a transformative shift toward personalized and continual monitoring, with wearable sensors playing a pivotal role. These devices, ranging from smartwatches to specialized medical wearables, have the potential to revolutionize patient care by providing real-time data and insights into various physiological parameters. Oxygen saturation, a critical parameter for respiratory health, can be accurately predicted from wearable sensor data using advanced machine learning techniques.

Oxygen saturation, commonly measured as SpO_2, represents the percentage of oxygenated hemoglobin in the blood. Maintaining optimal oxygen saturation levels is crucial for the proper functioning of vital organs and tissues. A deviation from the normal range can be indicative of respiratory disorders, cardiovascular issues, or other health complications. Traditional methods of monitoring oxygen saturation often involve periodic measurements using pulse oximeters, which can be cumbersome and do not provide continuous data. Wearable sensors offer a non-intrusive and continuous monitoring solution, allowing for timely detection of anomalies and proactive healthcare interventions.

Among the vital signs, pulse or heart rate emerges as a fundamental indicator of cardiovascular health. The rhythmic contraction and relaxation of the heart muscles, quantified in beats per minute (BPM), convey crucial information about the efficiency of the cardiovascular system. A deviation from the normal pulse rate may signify underlying health issues, underscoring the criticality of continuous pulse monitoring. Traditional methods of pulse monitoring involve sporadic measurements, often conducted manually or with the aid of medical devices. While effective in clinical settings, these methods fall short in providing a continuous and dynamic portrayal of an individual's pulse. Wearable sensors equipped with photoplethysmography (PPG) sensors, measuring blood volume changes in microvessels, present a revolutionary solution for continuous and non-intrusive pulse monitoring.

Respiration, a fundamental physiological process, serves as a vital indicator of an individual's overall health. Monitoring respiratory rate, depth, and patterns is crucial for the early detection of respiratory conditions, assessing cardiorespiratory fitness, and optimizing medical interventions. Traditional methods of respiratory monitoring often involve intrusive devices or cumbersome equipment, limiting their application in continuous and real-time monitoring scenarios. Ultra-Wideband (UWB) technology, initially developed for communication and radar applications, has found new horizons in healthcare.

UWB sensors operate across a broad frequency spectrum, enabling high precision in the localization and tracking of objects. The ability of UWB sensors to capture detailed temporal and spatial information makes them well-suited for monitoring dynamic physiological processes such as respiration.

UWB sensors utilize short-duration, low-power pulses transmitted across a wide frequency range. When these pulses encounter surfaces or objects, they generate echoes that are captured by the sensor. By analyzing the time delay and amplitude of these echoes, UWB sensors can precisely determine the distance and movement of objects in their vicinity. Applied to respiratory monitoring, UWB sensors detect subtle chest movements associated with inhalation and exhalation.

UWB sensors offer a contactless solution for respiratory monitoring, eliminating the need for physical attachments or uncomfortable devices. Placed in the environment or integrated into everyday objects, UWB sensors can capture respiratory data without direct contact with the individual, ensuring a non-intrusive and user-friendly experience. In home healthcare settings, UWB sensors contribute to Ambient Assisted Living (AAL) by continuously monitoring respiratory patterns. This is particularly valuable for aging populations or individuals with chronic respiratory conditions. UWB-enabled systems can detect deviations from normal respiratory patterns, triggering timely interventions or alerts to caregivers. In clinical settings, UWB sensors offer an innovative alternative to traditional respiratory monitoring devices. Patients can be monitored remotely, reducing the burden on healthcare infrastructure and providing healthcare professionals with real-time data. UWB sensors can be integrated into hospital beds, rooms, or wearable devices to enable seamless monitoring during hospital stays.

UWB sensors excel in providing high precision in localization, enabling accurate tracking of chest movements during respiration. This level of precision allows for detailed analysis of respiratory patterns, contributing to a more nuanced understanding of an individual's respiratory health. Advancements in UWB sensor technology have led to miniaturization, making it feasible to integrate these sensors into wearable devices. Wearable UWB sensors offer individuals the flexibility to incorporate respiratory monitoring into their daily lives, providing continuous insights without disrupting daily activities. The high data rate capabilities of UWB sensors facilitate real-time data analytics. This allows for immediate feedback on respiratory patterns, enabling timely interventions and personalized healthcare strategies. The integration of machine learning algorithms further enhances the interpretability of UWB-generated respiratory data. Figure 5.41 shows a schematic setup of real time monitoring of respiration using ambient UWB sensor and wearable pulse as well as oxygen saturation sensor.

5.4.1 LSTM for Prediction of Health Status

The integration of LSTM networks into predictive models for oxygen saturation from wearable sensor data represents a significant advancement in the field of predictive healthcare analytics. LSTMs, a type of recurrent neural network (RNN), are well-suited for handling sequential data, making them ideal for time-series analysis of physiological signals. This introduction aims to explore the rationale behind using LSTM networks in the context of

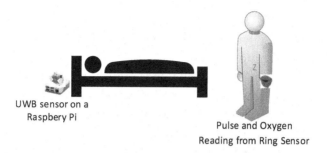

FIGURE 5.41 A schematic setup of real time monitoring of respiration using ambient UWB sensor and wearable pulse as well as oxygen saturation sensor.

oxygen saturation prediction, highlighting their strengths, challenges, and the potential impact on improving healthcare outcomes.

Wearable sensors have undergone a rapid evolution, transitioning from basic activity trackers to sophisticated health monitoring devices. These sensors leverage a combination of accelerometers, photoplethysmography (PPG) sensors, and other biometric sensors to capture a wealth of physiological data in real time. PPG sensors, in particular, play a crucial role in measuring oxygen saturation by analyzing the light absorption characteristics of blood. As individuals increasingly incorporate wearables into their daily lives, these devices become an invaluable source of continuous health data.

Continuous monitoring allows for a more comprehensive understanding of an individual's health status by capturing subtle changes that might go unnoticed in traditional episodic monitoring. Wearable sensors, equipped with the capability to measure oxygen saturation, offer a proactive approach to managing respiratory health and preventing complications.

Traditional machine learning models often struggle to effectively capture temporal dependencies in sequential data, a crucial aspect when dealing with physiological signals. LSTM networks, introduced to overcome the limitations of standard RNNs, excel at modeling long-range dependencies and have demonstrated superior performance in time-series analysis tasks.

LSTMs consist of memory cells that can retain information for extended periods, selectively updating and forgetting information based on the input data. This architecture allows LSTMs to capture complex temporal patterns, making them well-suited for tasks such as predicting oxygen saturation from time-varying sensor data. The ability to learn and remember patterns over extended time intervals is particularly advantageous in healthcare applications where subtle changes in physiological signals may precede clinically significant events.

While the integration of LSTM networks into predictive models for oxygen saturation holds great promise, it comes with its set of challenges. One primary concern is the need for large and diverse datasets to train these models effectively. The variability in physiological responses among individuals, the impact of different wearable sensor technologies, and the influence of external factors such as environmental conditions pose challenges in creating a robust and generalizable model.

5.4.2 ARIMA for Prediction of Health Status

ARIMA models, standing for Autoregressive Integrated Moving Average, are well-established tools for analyzing time-series data. These models are particularly adept at capturing the temporal dependencies and trends present in sequential data, making them suitable for physiological signal analysis. ARIMA models consist of autoregressive (AR), differencing (I), and moving average (MA) components, allowing them to account for seasonality, trends, and random fluctuations within a time series.

The autoregressive component of the ARIMA model focuses on capturing the relationship between a variable and its past values. In simpler terms, it assesses how previous observations influence the current one. The 'AR' parameter, denoted as 'p,' represents the number of past observations considered for predicting the future value. A higher 'p' signifies a more extensive dependency on past data. The autoregressive component is represented by:

$$y_t = \beta_0 + \beta_1 y_{t-1} + \beta_2 y_{t-2} + \ldots + \beta_{1p} y_{t-p} + \varepsilon_t$$

where y_t is the value of the time series at time t, β_0 is a constant term, $\beta_1, \beta_2 \ldots \beta_p$ are the autoregressive coefficients, and ε_t is the white noise or error term.

The differencing component of ARIMA addresses the issue of non-stationarity in time-series data. Non-stationarity occurs when the statistical properties of the data, such as mean and variance, change over time. The 'I' parameter, denoted as 'd,' represents the number of times differencing is applied to achieve stationarity. Differencing involves subtracting the current observation from its previous one, stabilizing the mean and removing trends.

The integrated component is represented by differencing the time series:

$$\Delta y_t = y_t - y_{t-1}$$

If differencing is performed d times to make the series stationary, then the model is ARIMA(p,d,q). The moving average component of ARIMA focuses on modeling the relationship between a variable and a stochastic term derived from past observations. This component helps capture short-term fluctuations or noise in the data. The 'MA' parameter, denoted as 'q,' represents the number of past stochastic terms considered in predicting the future value. Similar to the 'p' parameter, a higher 'q' indicates a more substantial reliance on recent stochastic terms. The moving average component is represented by:

$$y_t = \beta_0 + \varepsilon_t + \theta_1 \varepsilon_{t-1} + \theta_2 \varepsilon_{t-2} + \ldots + \theta_q \varepsilon_{t-q}$$

where $\theta_1, \theta_2, \theta_q$ are the moving average coefficients and ε_t is the white noise or error term.

The ARIMA model combines these three components to create a mathematical representation that can be used for forecasting. The general notation for an ARIMA model is represented as ARIMA(p, d, q), where 'p,' 'd,' and 'q' denote the respective AR, differencing, and MA parameters. For example, an ARIMA(2, 1, 1) model signifies an autoregressive order of 2, a differencing order of 1, and a moving average order of 1. To create an ARIMA model, the first step involves assessing the stationarity of the time-series data. If the data is non-stationary, differencing is applied until stationarity is achieved. Once the data is stationary, the model parameters 'p' and 'q' are determined through a process known as model identification, often involving the analysis of autocorrelation and partial autocorrelation functions.

The next steps involve model estimation and diagnostics. The model is fitted to the historical data, and the residuals are analyzed to ensure that they exhibit no discernible patterns or trends. If necessary, adjustments are made to the model parameters to improve its performance. Combining the autoregressive, integrated, and moving average components, the ARIMA model equation is given by:

$$\Delta^d y_t = \beta_0 + \beta_1 \Delta^d y_{t-1} + \beta_2 \Delta^d y_{t-2} + \ldots + \beta_p \Delta^d y_{t-p} + \varepsilon_t + \theta_1 \varepsilon_{t-1} + \theta_2 \varepsilon_{t-2} + \ldots + \theta_q \varepsilon_{t-q}$$

where $\Delta^d y_t$ represents the dth order differenced series. In these equations, y_t represents the observed values of the time series at time t, and ε_t represents the white noise or error term at time t. The coefficients (β_0, β_1, ..., β_p, θ_1, ..., θ_q) are parameters estimated during the modeling process.

ARIMA models are versatile and can be applied to a wide range of time-series data, making them a valuable tool in various fields. The interpretability of ARIMA models allows users to understand the impact of past observations and trends on future predictions. This transparency is crucial in fields where decision-making relies on a clear understanding of the model's behavior. ARIMA models excel in short-term forecasting, providing accurate predictions for time intervals within the scope of the historical data. ARIMA models can be sensitive to outliers or extreme values in the data. Outliers may disproportionately influence the model's performance, necessitating careful preprocessing. ARIMA models assume a linear relationship between past and future observations. In cases where non-linear relationships exist, alternative modeling techniques may be more suitable. ARIMA models may exhibit limitations when applied to long-term forecasting, as they rely heavily on past observations and may not capture complex, evolving patterns.

In the context of predicting oxygen saturation from wearable sensor data, ARIMA models can be tailored to capture the inherent patterns and variations present in the time-series measurements. The adaptability of ARIMA models to changes in the data over time makes them suitable for handling the dynamic nature of physiological signals, allowing for accurate predictions and early detection of potential health issues. While ARIMA models offer a powerful approach to time-series analysis, they are not without challenges. These models assume stationarity in the data, and adapting them to handle non-stationary physiological signals can be complex. Moreover, the accuracy of ARIMA predictions is contingent on the availability of sufficient historical data and the accurate identification of model parameters. The heterogeneity in physiological responses among individuals and the impact of different wearable sensor technologies also pose challenges in developing robust and generalizable ARIMA models for predicting oxygen saturation.

The successful application of ARIMA and LSTM models for predicting oxygen saturation from wearable sensor data holds the potential to significantly impact healthcare outcomes.

Timely predictions allow for proactive healthcare interventions, enabling healthcare providers to address respiratory issues promptly and prevent complications. The continuous monitoring facilitated by wearable sensors, in conjunction with ARIMA predictions, provides a holistic and real-time perspective on an individual's health status. Remote patient monitoring, empowered by LSTM and ARIMA-based predictive analytics, can enhance healthcare delivery by reducing the need for frequent hospital visits and emergency room admissions. Individuals, equipped with the knowledge gained from continuous monitoring, can actively participate in managing their health and making informed decisions regarding lifestyle adjustments. This patient-centric approach aligns with the broader goals of personalized and preventive healthcare. Moreover, the continuous feedback loop established through wearable sensors and LSTM and ARIMA-based predictions fosters a more patient-centric approach to healthcare. Individuals gain greater awareness of their health status, enabling them to make informed lifestyle choices and adhere to preventive measures. This shift toward proactive and personalized healthcare aligns with the broader goal of leveraging technology to transform the healthcare landscape.

5.4.3 Case Study of Oxygen Saturation, Pulse, and Respiration Prediction

For the case studies of oxygen saturation, pulse, and respiration prediction using machine learning, the data is recorded by author himself to show the examples. However, any other floating number data sequences can be used for prediction. LSTM code for oxygen saturation prediction is as follows and Figure 5.42 shows LSTM prediction of oxygen saturation where dark points are the training data prediction, and light points are testing data prediction. The dataset used for oxygen saturation and pulse can be obtained from https://github.com/Zia-Uddin-81/Book_SHA_ML_Python/blob/main/oxygen_pulse.csv. The dataset for respiration can be obtained from https://github.com/Zia-Uddin-81/Book_SHA_ML_Python/blob/main/Respiration.csv.

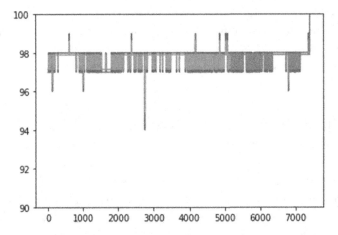

FIGURE 5.42 LSTM prediction of oxygen saturation where dark part is training data prediction and light part is testing data prediction.

```python
import numpy as np
import matplotlib.pyplot as plt
from pandas import read_csv
import math
import tensorflow as tf
from tensorflow.keras.models import Sequential
from tensorflow.keras.layers import Dense
from tensorflow.keras.layers import LSTM
from sklearn.preprocessing import MinMaxScaler
from sklearn.metrics import mean_squared_error
# convert an array of values into a dataset matrix

def create _ dataset(dataset, window _ size=1):
    dataX, dataY = [], []
    for i in range(len(dataset)-window_size-1):
        a = dataset[i:(i+window_size), 0]
        dataX.append(a)
        dataY.append(dataset[i + window_size, 0])
    return np.array(dataX), np.array(dataY)

dataframe = read_csv('oxygen_pulse.csv', usecols=[1],
engine='python')

dataset = dataframe.values
dataset = dataset.astype('float32')

scaler = MinMaxScaler(feature _ range=(0, 1))
dataset = scaler.fit_transform(dataset)

# split into train and test sets
train_size = int(len(dataset) * 0.70)
test_size = len(dataset) - train_size
train, test = dataset[0:train_size,:],
dataset[train_size:len(dataset),:]

# reshape into X=t and Y=t+1
window_size = 1
trainX, trainY = create_dataset(train, window_size)
testX, testY = create_dataset(test, window_size)

# reshape input to be [samples, time steps, features]
trainX = np.reshape(trainX, (trainX.shape[0], 1, trainX.shape[1]))
testX = np.reshape(testX, (testX.shape[0], 1, testX.shape[1]))

model = Sequential()
model.add(LSTM(10, input_shape=(1, window_size)))
model.add(Dense(1))
model.compile(loss='mean_squared_error', optimizer='adam')
model.fit(trainX, trainY, epochs=100, batch_size=1, verbose=2)

# make predictions
trainPredict = model.predict(trainX)
```

```
testPredict = model.predict(testX)
trainPredict = scaler.inverse_transform(trainPredict)
trainY = scaler.inverse_transform([trainY])
testPredict = scaler.inverse_transform(testPredict)
testY = scaler.inverse_transform([testY])

# calculate root mean squared error
trainScore = np.sqrt(mean_squared_error(trainY[0],
trainPredict[:,0]))
print('Train Score: %.2f RMSE' % (trainScore))
testScore = np.sqrt(mean_squared_error(testY[0], testPredict[:,0]))
print('Test Score: %.2f RMSE' % (testScore))

# shift train predictions for plotting
# invert predictions
trainPredictPlot = np.empty_like(dataset)
trainPredictPlot[:, :] = np.nan
trainPredictPlot[window_size:len(trainPredict)+window_size, :] =
trainPredict

# shift test predictions for plotting
testPredictPlot = np.empty_like(dataset)
testPredictPlot[:, :] = np.nan
testPredictPlot[len(trainPredict)+(window_size*2)+1:len
(dataset)-1, :] = testPredict

# plot baseline and predictions
plt.plot(scaler.inverse_transform(dataset))
plt.plot(trainPredictPlot)
plt.plot(testPredictPlot)
plt.ylim(90, 100)
plt.figure(figsize=(6,4))
plt.show()
```

Figure 5.43 shows the model summary and Figure 5.44 ARIMA prediction of oxygen saturation where dark points are the test data and light points are predictions of that data. ARIMA code is as follows:

```
import numpy as np
import matplotlib.pyplot as plt
from pandas import read_csv
import math
from sklearn.metrics import mean_squared_error
import warnings
import itertools
from pandas import datetime
from pandas import read_csv
from pandas import DataFrame
from statsmodels.tsa.arima.model import ARIMA
```

```
                          SARIMAX Results
================================================================================
Dep. Variable:                     y   No. Observations:               7414
Model:                ARIMA(5, 1, 0)   Log Likelihood             -15058.636
Date:               Fri, 05 Jan 2024   AIC                         30129.272
Time:                       23:24:14   BIC                         30170.738
Sample:                            0   HQIC                        30143.520
                              - 7414
Covariance Type:                 opg
================================================================================
                 coef    std err          z      P>|z|      [0.025      0.975]
--------------------------------------------------------------------------------
ar.L1         -0.0043      0.032     -0.132      0.895      -0.068       0.059
ar.L2         -0.1779      0.348     -0.511      0.610      -0.861       0.505
ar.L3         -0.1534      0.353     -0.435      0.664      -0.845       0.539
ar.L4         -0.1154      0.368     -0.314      0.754      -0.836       0.606
ar.L5         -0.1101      0.362     -0.304      0.761      -0.820       0.600
sigma2         3.4037      0.001   3620.679      0.000       3.402       3.406
================================================================================
Ljung-Box (Q):                  1.13   Jarque-Bera (JB):    15446468056.02
Prob(Q):                        1.00   Prob(JB):                      0.00
Heteroskedasticity (H):       160.83   Skew:                         83.12
Prob(H) (two-sided):            0.00   Kurtosis:                   7072.74
================================================================================
```

FIGURE 5.43   SARIMAX model summary.

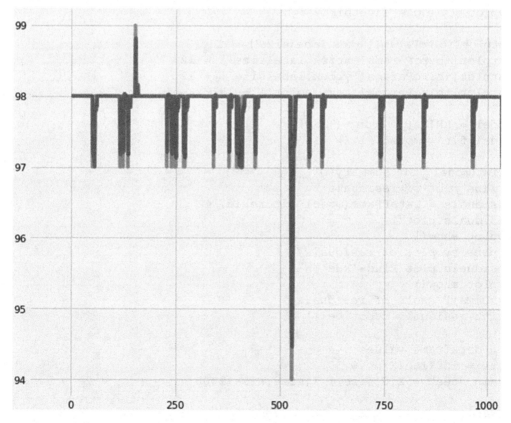

FIGURE 5.44   ARIMA prediction of oxygen saturation where dark part is training data prediction and light part is testing data prediction.

```
from matplotlib import pyplot
import matplotlib
import pandas as pd
from math import sqrt

# convert an array of values into a dataset matrix

def create_dataset(dataset):
    dataX, dataY = [], []
    for i in range(len(dataset)):
        a = dataset[i:(i+1), 0]
        dataX.append(a)
        dataY.append(dataset[i + 1, 0])
    return np.array(dataX), np.array(dataY)

dataframe = read_csv('oxygen_pulse.csv', usecols=[1], engine='python')

dataset = dataframe.values
dataset = dataset.astype('float32')

y=dataset

pyplot.style.use('fivethirtyeight')

matplotlib.rcParams['axes.labelsize'] = 14
matplotlib.rcParams['xtick.labelsize'] = 12
matplotlib.rcParams['ytick.labelsize'] = 12
matplotlib.rcParams['text.color'] = 'k'

model = ARIMA(y, order=(5,1,0))
model_fit = model.fit()

print(model_fit.summary())
# line plot of residuals
residuals = DataFrame(model_fit.resid)
residuals.plot()
pyplot.show()
# density plot of residuals
residuals.plot(kind='kde')
pyplot.show()
# summary stats of residuals
print(residuals.describe())

X = dataframe.values
size = int(len(X) * 0.30)
train, test = X[0:size], X[size:size+2000]

#train, test = X[0:size], X[size:len(X)]
history = [x for x in train]
predictions = list()
```

```
# walk-forward validation
for t in range(len(test)):
    model = ARIMA(history, order=(5,1,0))
    model_fit = model.fit()
    output = model_fit.forecast()
    yhat = output[0]
    predictions.append(yhat)
    obs = test[t]
    history.append(obs)

rmse = sqrt(mean _ squared _ error(test, predictions))
print('Test RMSE: %.3f' % rmse)

# plot forecasts against actual outcomes
pyplot.plot(test)
pyplot.plot(predictions, color='red')
pyplot.show()
```

Using the same code but just only changing the dataset representing pulse and respiration, Figures 5.45–5.48 obtained.

5.4.4 Sleep Quality Analysis

Sleep is a fundamental aspect of our well-being, intricately tied to various factors such as sleep duration, quality, and the choices we make in our daily lives. It plays a vital role in our overall health and functionality, influencing both physical and mental well-being. Understanding the interconnections between our sleep patterns, lifestyle choices, and health outcomes is crucial for promoting optimal health.

Our daily choices significantly impact the quality of our sleep. Irregular sleep schedules, poor dietary habits, sedentary lifestyles, and heightened stress levels can disrupt

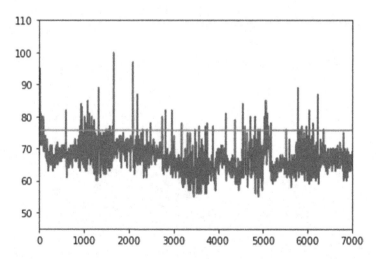

FIGURE 5.45   LSTM prediction of pulse where dark part is training data prediction and light part is testing data prediction.

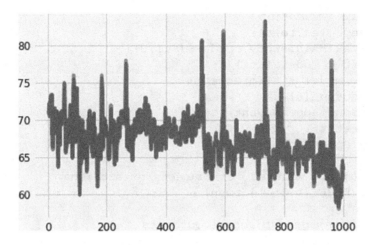

FIGURE 5.46   ARIMA prediction of pulse where dark part is training data prediction and light part is testing data prediction.

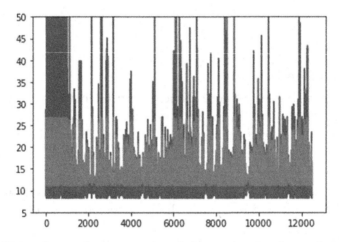

FIGURE 5.47   LSTM prediction of respiration where dark part is training data prediction and light part is testing data prediction.

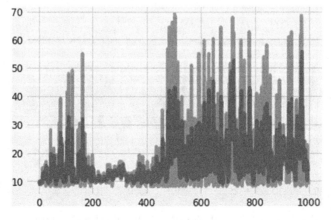

FIGURE 5.48   ARIMA prediction of respiration where dark part is training data prediction and light part is testing data prediction.

our sleep patterns, leading to a range of health issues. On the contrary, cultivating positive habits, maintaining a healthy diet, incorporating regular physical activity, and managing stress contribute to better sleep quality and overall well-being.

In the domain of sleep disorders, sleep apnea stands out as a common condition characterized by pauses in breathing during sleep. Early detection and intervention are essential for effectively managing sleep apnea and mitigating potential health complications. This is where the integration of machine learning into sleep health becomes particularly promising.

Machine learning, with its capacity to analyze vast and diverse datasets, offers an innovative approach to predicting sleep disorders, specifically sleep apnea. By leveraging comprehensive datasets that include information related to sleep duration, snoring patterns, physical activity levels, body mass index (BMI), and more, machine learning algorithms can discern intricate patterns and subtle indicators associated with the risk of sleep apnea.

The process involves extracting meaningful features from the data, such as the intensity of snoring or the duration of sleep, which serve as inputs for the machine learning algorithms. Through supervised learning techniques, the models are trained on historical data that includes instances of sleep apnea and corresponding sleep health and lifestyle attributes. This training enables the model to learn patterns indicative of sleep apnea risk.

Once trained, the machine learning model can then make predictions on new and unseen data. By inputting relevant sleep health and lifestyle information, the model assesses the likelihood of sleep apnea. Continuous monitoring and updates allow for the refinement of the model over time, adapting to changing sleep patterns and lifestyle choices, ultimately enhancing its predictive capabilities.

Looking ahead, the future holds the promise of a more personalized approach to sleep health. The convergence between sleep science, lifestyle insights, and machine learning offers a pathway for individuals to proactively manage their sleep health. As research and technology progress, this fusion opens new possibilities for understanding, predicting, and addressing sleep-related challenges, ultimately contributing to improved overall well-being.

5.4.5 Case Study of Sleep Quality Analysis

For prediction of the presence of sleep apnea in a person, a small dataset is used. The dataset is called *Sleep Health and Lifestyle* Dataset and collected from https://www.kaggle.com/datasets/uom190346a/sleep-health-and-lifestyle-dataset. The dataset related to sleep and daily habits, known as the Sleep Health and Lifestyle Dataset, is comprised of 400 rows and 13 columns, providing a comprehensive array of variables. These variables encompass information such as gender, age, occupation, sleep duration, sleep quality, physical activity level, stress levels, BMI category, blood pressure, heart rate, daily steps, and the presence or absence of sleep disorders. For our analysis, we will be utilizing the "Sleep_health_and_lifestyle_dataset.csv" database, which has been made accessible for our purposes. Below, you will find an examination of the data, the processing steps applied to it, and the utilization of machine learning classification models to achieve our objectives.

Let's import the library first as

```
import pandas as pd
import numpy as np
import matplotlib.pyplot as plt
import seaborn as sns
import plotly.express as px
from sklearn.metrics import accuracy_score, confusion_matrix,
classification_report
from sklearn.tree import DecisionTreeClassifier
from sklearn.metrics import r2_score
from sklearn.metrics import mean_absolute_error, mean_squared_error
from sklearn.model_selection import GridSearchCV
from sklearn.model_selection import RandomizedSearchCV
from sklearn.preprocessing import LabelEncoder
from tensorflow.keras.models import Sequential
from tensorflow.keras.layers import Dense
from tensorflow.keras.layers import LSTM
from tensorflow.keras.preprocessing import sequence
```

Then load the dataset in dataframe as

```
df = pd.read_csv('./Sleep_health_and_lifestyle_dataset.csv', sep = ',')
```

By running *df.head()*, we can see the head rows of the dataset as bellow in Table 5.7.

In the dataset, there are following columns or attributes.

- Person ID: An identifier assigned to each individual.

- Gender: The biological sex of the person (Male/Female).

- Age: The age of the person in years.

- Occupation: The occupation or profession of the person.

- Sleep Duration (hours): The total number of hours the person sleeps per day.

- Quality of Sleep: A subjective assessment of sleep quality, rated on a scale from 1 to 10.

- Physical Activity Level (minutes/day): The amount of time the person dedicates to physical activity each day.

- Stress Level (scale: 1–10): A subjective evaluation of the stress level experienced by the person, ranging from 1 to 10.

- BMI Category: The Body Mass Index (BMI) category of the person, such as Underweight, Normal, or Overweight.

- Blood Pressure (systolic/diastolic): The recorded blood pressure of the person, presented as systolic pressure over diastolic pressure.

- Heart Rate (bpm): The resting heart rate of the person, measured in beats per minute.

- Daily Steps: The total count of steps taken by the person on a daily basis.

- Sleep Disorder: Indicates whether the person has a sleep disorder (None, Insomnia, Sleep Apnea).

TABLE 5.7 Dataset Head of Sleep Quality

	Person ID	Gender	Age	Occupation	Sleep Duration	Quality of Sleep	Physical Activity Level	Stress Level	BMI Category	Blood Pressure	Heart Rate	Daily Steps	Sleep Disorder
0	1	Male	27	Software Engineer	6.1	6	42	6	Overweight	126/83	77	4200	None
1	2	Malo	28	Doctor	6.2	6	60	8	Normal	125/80	75	10000	None
2	3	Male	28	Doctor	62	6	60	8	Normal	125/80	75	10000	None
3	4	Malo	28	Sales Representative	5.9	4	30	8	Obeso	140/90	85	3000	Sleep Apnea
4	5	Male	28	Sales Representative	59	4	30	8	Obese	140/90	85	3000	Sleep Apnea

TABLE 5.8   Dataset Description of Sleep Quality

	Person ID	Age	Sleep Duration	Quality of Sleep	Physical Activity Level	Stress Level	Heart Rate	Daily Steps
Count	374.000000	374.000000	374.000000	374.000000	374.000000	374.000000	374.000000	374.000000
Mean	187.500000	42.184492	7.132086	7.312834	59.171123	5.385027	70.165775	6816.844920
Std	108.108742	8.673133	0.795657	1.196956	20.830804	1.774526	4.135676	1617.915679
Min	1.000000	27.000000	5.800000	4.000000	30.000000	3.000000	65.000000	3000.000000
25%	94.250000	35.250000	6.400000	6.000000	45.000000	4.000000	68.000000	5600.000000
50%	187.500000	43.000000	7.200000	7.000000	60.000000	5.000000	70.000000	7000.000000
75%	280.750000	50.000000	7.800000	8.000000	75.000000	7.000000	72.000000	8000.000000
Max	374.000000	59.000000	8.500000	9.000000	90.000000	8.000000	86.000000	10000.000000

The statement *df.describe()* generates output as in Table 5.8.

The data correlation can be found as follows. The output is shown in Figure 5.49.

```
corr = df.corr()
plt.figure(figsize = (15,6))
sns.heatmap(corr, annot = True, cmap = 'crest', annot_kws={"size":
12})
```

The other attribute feature relevance with respect to sleep disorder can be obtained as follows and Figure 5.50 shows the output boxplots.

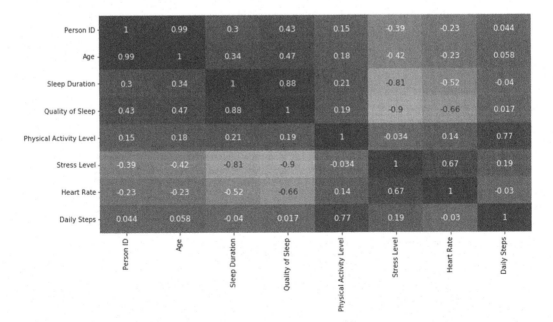

FIGURE 5.49   Seaborn heatmap sleep quality data correlation.

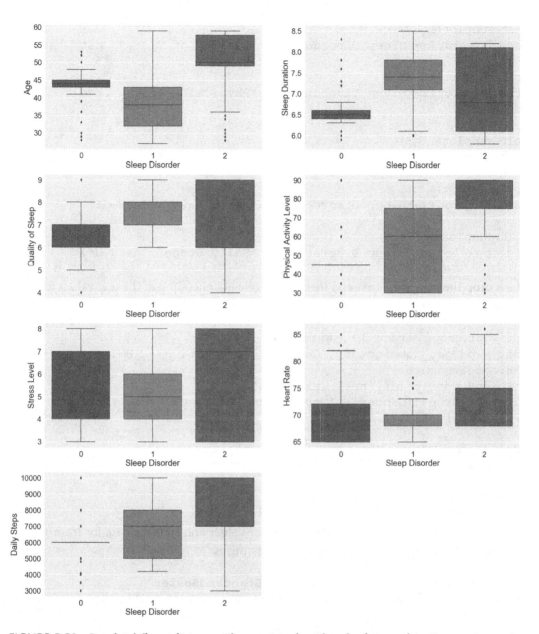

FIGURE 5.50 Boxplot different features with respect to sleep disorder feature where 0 means insomnia, 1 none, and 2 sleep apneas.

```
plt.figure(figsize = (25, 20))
plt.suptitle("Analysis Of Variable Sleep
Disorder",fontweight="bold", fontsize=20)

plt.subplot(4,2,1)
sns.boxplot(x="Sleep Disorder", y="Age", data=df)

plt.subplot(4,2,2)
sns.boxplot(x="Sleep Disorder", y="Sleep Duration", data=df)
```

```
plt.subplot(4,2,3)
sns.boxplot(x="Sleep Disorder", y="Quality of Sleep", dat    a=df)

plt.subplot(4,2,4)
sns.boxplot(x="Sleep Disorder", y="Physical Activity Level",
data=df)

plt.subplot(4,2,5)
sns.boxplot(x="Sleep Disorder", y="Stress Level", data=df)

plt.subplot(4,2,6)
sns.boxplot(x="Sleep Disorder", y="Heart Rate", data=df)

plt.subplot(4,2,7)
sns.boxplot(x="Sleep Disorder", y="Daily Steps", data=df)
```

Let's drop the person ID first and then do the one hot encoding of the text values to make numeric values and obtain X and y variables as

```
df = df.drop('Person ID', axis = 1)
hot = pd.get_dummies(df[['Gender', 'Occupation', 'BMI Category',
'Blood Pressure']])
df = pd.concat([df, hot], axis = 1)
df = df.drop(['Gender', 'Occupation', 'BMI Category', 'Blood
Pressure'], axis = 1)

X = df.drop('Sleep Disorder', axis = 1)
X = X.values

y = df['Sleep Disorder']
```

Then, let us normalize the X by standard scalar values and split the data for training and testing as 70% data for training and 30% for testing as:

```
from sklearn.preprocessing import StandardScaler
from sklearn.model_selection import train_test_split
scaler = StandardScaler()
X_normalized = scaler.fit_transform(X)
X_train, X_test, y_train, y_test = train_test_split(X_normalized,
y, test_size = 0.3, random_state = 0)
```

Let us define a function to plot confusion matrix and show the accuracy score.

```
def plot_confusion_matrix(y_test, y_preds):
    cm = confusion_matrix(y_test, y_preds)
    classes = ['Insomnia', 'None', 'Sleep Apnea']
    ax = sns.heatmap(cm, cbar=False, cmap="Blues", annot=True,
annot_kws={"size": 18}, fmt='g', xticklabels=classes,
yticklabels=classes)
  print(accuracy_score(y_test, y_preds))
```

Then let us run the decision tree as

```
decision _ tree = DecisionTreeClassifier(criterion = 'entropy', min _
samples _ split = 6, max _ depth= 6, random _ state=0)
decision_tree.fit(X_train, y_train)
y_preds = decision_tree.predict(X_test)
plot_confusion_matrix(y_test, y_preds)
```

The Decision Tree classifier accuracy is 0.89 and the output confusion matrix is shown in Figure 5.51.

The seaborn plot is the same code as Decision Trees for other classifiers and hence, following code is to apply Random Forest classification.

```
from sklearn.ensemble import RandomForestClassifier
random_forest = RandomForestClassifier(n_estimators = 100, min_
samples_split = 5, max_depth= 5,  criterion = 'gini', random_state = 0)
random_forest.fit(X_train, y_train)
y_preds = random_forest.predict(X_test)
plot_confusion_matrix(y_test, y_preds)
```

The Random Forest classifier accuracy is 0.90 and the output confusion matrix is shown in Figure 5.52.

The K-nearest neighbor (KNN) classifier was applied as

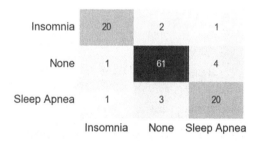

FIGURE 5.51   Confusion matrix sleep quality using Decision Trees classifier.

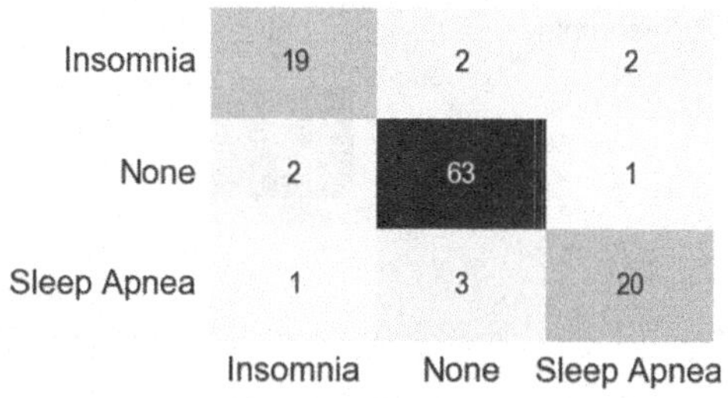

FIGURE 5.52   Confusion matrix sleep quality using random forest classifier.

```
from sklearn.neighbors import KNeighborsClassifier
knn = KNeighborsClassifier(n_neighbors = 5, metric = 'minkowski', p = 2)
knn.fit(X_train, y_train)
y_preds = knn.predict(X_test)
plot_confusion_matrix(y_test, y_preds)
```

The KNN classifier accuracy is 0.88 and the output confusion matrix is shown in Figure 5.53.

The logistic regression can be applied as:

```
from sklearn.linear_model import LogisticRegression
logistic = LogisticRegression(random_state = 1, max_iter=10000)
logistic.fit(X_train, y_train)
y_preds = logistic.predict(X_test)
plot_confusion_matrix(y_test, y_preds)
```

The logistic regression classifier accuracy is 0.92 and the output confusion matrix is shown in Figure 5.54.

The AdaBoost code in this regard was as follows.

```
from sklearn.ensemble import AdaBoostClassifier
ada_boost = AdaBoostClassifier(n_estimators = 500, learning_rate = 0.02, random_state = 0)
ada_boost.fit(X_train, y_train)
y_preds = ada_boost.predict(X_test)
plot_confusion_matrix(y_test, y_preds)
```

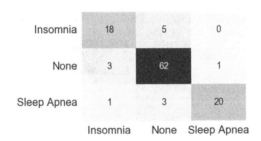

FIGURE 5.53   Confusion matrix sleep quality using k nearest neighbor classifier.

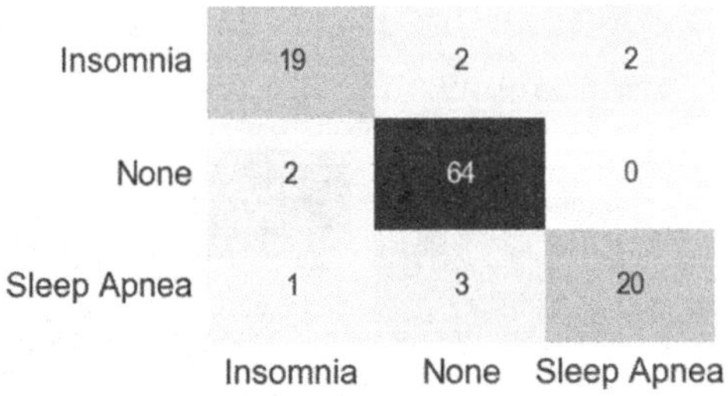

FIGURE 5.54   Confusion matrix sleep quality using logistic regression classifier.

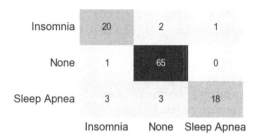

FIGURE 5.55   Confusion matrix sleep quality using AdaBoost classifier.

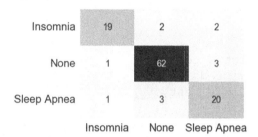

FIGURE 5.56   Confusion matrix sleep quality using GradientBoost classifier.

The AdaBoost classifier accuracy is 0.91 and the output confusion matrix is shown in Figure 5.55.

The GradientBoost was applied as below.

```
from sklearn.ensemble import GradientBoostingClassifier
model = GradientBoostingClassifier(n_estimators = 500, learning_
rate =  0.02)
model.fit(X_train, y_train)
y_preds = model.predict(X_test)
plot_confusion_matrix(y_test, y_preds)
```

The GradientBoost classifier accuracy is 0.89 and the output confusion matrix is shown in Figure 5.56.

To apply method LSTM, the text categories of sleep disorder column was numerically represented from 0 to 2. It was applied as bellow.

```
y = df['Sleep Disorder']
y.replace({'Insomnia':0, 'None':1, 'Sleep Apnea':2}, inplace=True)

X_standard =X_standard.reshape(374,1,49)
X_train, X_test, y_train, y_test = train_test_split(X_standard, y,
test_size = 0.3, random_state = 0)
# create and fit the LSTM network
model = Sequential()
model.add(LSTM(10, input_shape=(1,49)))
model.add(Dense(3))
```

```
model.compile(loss='mean_squared_error', optimizer='adam')
history = model.fit(X_train , y_train, epochs=500, batch_size=10,
verbose=2)

import matplotlib.pyplot as plt
plt.plot(history.history['loss'], label='train_loss')
#plt.plot(history.history['val_loss'], label='val_loss')
plt.title('Training  Loss')
plt.xlabel('Epoch')
plt.ylabel('Loss')
plt.legend()
plt.show()

import numpy as np
preds = model.predict(X_test)
y_preds = np.argmax(preds , axis = 1 )
plot_confusion_matrix(y_test, y_preds)
```

That generates the accuracy of only 0.33 with 500 epoch for training. The following figure shows the epoch versus loss plot for training. LSTM code followed by the confusion matrix drawn using seaborn module shown in the first experiment. Figure 5.57 shows the epoch versus loss plot of the LSTM model. Figure 5.58 shows the confusion matrix using LSTM. Table 5.9 summarizes the accuracies of different machine learning algorithms where deep learning model LSTM shows the lowest accuracy though but further parameter and epoch tuning should improve its results

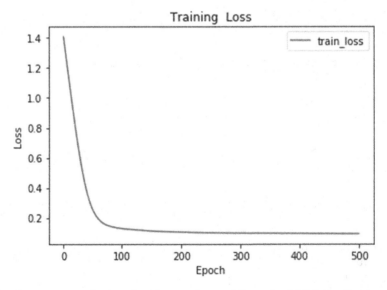

FIGURE 5.57   Loss versus epochs regarding sleep quality modeling using LSTM classifier.

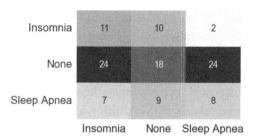

FIGURE 5.58   Confusion matrix sleep quality using LSTM classifier.

TABLE 5.9   Accuracies of Different Machine Learning
Approaches Codes on Sleep Quality Dataset

Approach	Accuracy
Decision Trees	0.89
Random Forest	0.90
KNN	0.88
Logistic Regression	0.92
AdaBoost	0.91
GradientBoost	0.89
LSTM	0.33

5.5 SYNTHETIC DATA GENERATION

The digital age has led us by an unprecedented amount of data, emphasizing the importance of strong and varied datasets for various applications [64, 65]. In machine learning,
artificial intelligence, and data analytics, the quality and quantity of training data play a
pivotal role in the efficacy of models. However, challenges such as data scarcity, privacy
concerns, and ethical considerations often hinder the acquisition of real-world datasets
that are sufficiently representative and comprehensive. Synthetic data generation algorithms have emerged as a transformative solution to overcome these challenges, offering
the ability to create artificial datasets that exhibit statistical properties similar to authentic
data. The motivation for exploring synthetic data generation algorithms is rooted in the
increasing demand for large and varied datasets. Real-world datasets are often limited,
especially in sensitive domains where data privacy is crucial. Synthetic data generation
algorithms address this gap by providing a means to generate artificial datasets that mirror the statistical characteristics of real-world data. This capability becomes particularly
crucial in scenarios where collecting additional authentic data is impractical, expensive, or
ethically challenging.

The evolution of synthetic data generation algorithms traces a journey from early heu-
ristic methods to sophisticated, model-driven approaches used today. Early attempts often
relied on simple heuristics, lacking the capacity to capture intricate relationships within
real-world datasets. The landscape has shifted with advanced machine learning techniques,
including Generative Adversarial Networks (GANs), Variational Autoencoders (VAEs),

and the Synthetic Data Vault (SDV). In particular, SDV stands out as a contemporary solution, incorporating various generative models and statistical techniques. SDV learns the underlying structure and patterns from existing real-world data, enabling the generation of synthetic datasets with high fidelity. SDV represents a significant advancement, replicating the complexity and diversity present in authentic datasets. By understanding the underlying distributions and relationships within real data, SDV facilitates the creation of synthetic datasets essential for training and testing machine learning models. The applications of synthetic data generation algorithms, including SDV, span across diverse domains. In healthcare, synthetic datasets aid in developing models for medical imaging and diagnostics. In finance, they assist in risk assessment and fraud detection. Synthetic data is crucial where sharing real data raises privacy concerns.

Despite the promising potential of synthetic data generation algorithms, challenges persist. Ensuring the quality and diversity of synthetic datasets, understanding the implications of biased generation, and developing robust evaluation metrics are critical concerns. Future research may address these challenges, explore novel generative models, and establish standardized practices for synthetic data generation. So, synthetic data generation algorithms, with SDV as a representative, offer a solution to challenges associated with data availability, privacy, and diversity. Creating realistic synthetic datasets advances machine learning, artificial intelligence, and data analytics. This introduction sets the groundwork for further exploration in synthetic data generation, emphasizing SDV's pivotal role in shaping the future of data-driven applications.

In the healthcare sector, vital signs such as heart rate, pulse, oxygen saturation, and respirations serve as critical parameters that reflect an individual's physiological well-being. Harnessing the power of synthetic data in monitoring these vital signs has emerged as a game-changer, offering solutions to data privacy concerns, enabling robust model training, and advancing medical diagnostics.

Real-world health data, especially pertaining to vital signs, is inherently sensitive and laden with privacy concerns. Synthetic data steps in as a privacy-conscious alternative, allowing the creation of artificial datasets that mirror the statistical properties of real health data without compromising individual privacy. This is particularly significant in complying with stringent healthcare regulations, ensuring ethical data usage for research and development. Vital sign monitoring demands diverse and realistic datasets for training models that can adapt to various scenarios. Synthetic data proves invaluable by augmenting limited real-world datasets, providing a broader spectrum of scenarios, patient profiles, and medical conditions. This augmentation enhances the adaptability and generalization capabilities of machine learning models, fostering the development of more accurate and reliable predictive models for vital sign monitoring. In the domain of medical diagnostics, synthetic data plays a pivotal role in enhancing the analysis of vital signs. By generating synthetic datasets that accurately represent variations in heart rate, pulse, oxygen saturation, and respirations, researchers can train machine learning models to interpret and diagnose abnormalities. This capability becomes particularly crucial in the early detection of health issues, facilitating timely interventions and improving patient outcomes.

Following is a sample code to generate respiration data discussed in previous subsection.

```
# # Getting Started with Synthetic Data Generation using SDV Python
Library

#Import Required Libraries
import pandas as pd
from sdv.metadata import SingleTableMetadata
from sdv.single_table import GaussianCopulaSynthesizer

# Read the original data
sample = pd.read_csv('./Respiration.csv', index_col=0)

# Generate metadata
metadata = SingleTableMetadata()
metadata.detect_from_dataframe(data=sample)

# Apply GaussianCopulaSynthesizer to generate synthetic data
synthesizer = GaussianCopulaSynthesizer(metadata)
synthesizer.fit(sample)
synthetic_data = synthesizer.sample(num_rows=5000)
synthetic_data.index.name = 'id'

# Draw the frequency of the original and synthetic data to evaluate
from sdv.evaluation.single_table import get_column_plot
fig = get_column_plot(
    real_data=sample,
    synthetic_data=synthetic_data,
    column_name='Respirations',
    metadata=metadata
)
fig.show()
#plot some samples from real  and synthetic data
plt.figure(figsize=(10,4))
plt.plot(real_data_respiration[100:500], 'r', label='Real Data
Samples')
plt.plot(synthetic_data_respiration[100:500], 'b',
label='Synthetic Data Samples')
plt.ylim(8,60)
plt.legend()
plt.show()
```

The code generates following Figure 5.59, which shows similar trends of synthetic and original data in terms of frequencies. Figure 5.60 shows some samples of real and synthetic data where synthetic data seems to be generated in the similar range of real data, without overlapping each other.

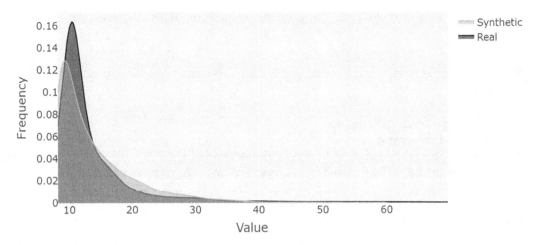

FIGURE 5.59   Synthetic data versus original data of respirations.

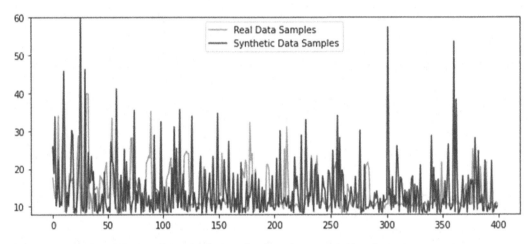

FIGURE 5.60   Some sequential samples from real and synthetic respiration data.

5.6 CONCLUSION

This chapter has explored diverse data, datasets, and experimental findings related to assisted living environments based on wearable and ambient sensors. Assisted living can utilize public datasets, which encompass information from various sources, to model different events (e.g., behavior, environment, and health status) using diverse machine learning algorithms. A considerable concern revolves around delivering healthcare to individuals at home, in clinics, or in hospitals, as unforeseen circumstances may negatively impact their health. To improve healthcare and independent living services in a cost-effective and dependable manner, it is crucial to incorporate technologies aiding people. Real-time monitoring of residents' environment and activities is essential in assisted care applications through an event-driven system. To identify current practices for future research directions, it is necessary to explore the literature on user care systems, an emerging area of research and development. Consequently, this book seeks to offer a comprehensive review of various smart user care systems, covering data sources, features, machine learning, and explainable artificial intelligence.

To inspire readers in the field, practical insights into the implementation of machine learning applications using sensor data have also been discussed, accompanied by examples primarily coded in Python to illustrate the concepts. The objective of this research was to gain knowledge about sensor-based user monitoring technologies in home environments. Research efforts have been made to adopt these technologies with the aim of facilitating independent living, and references will be provided for their use. While research on user monitoring technologies in assisted living is widespread, most of it comprises limited-scale studies, prompting the creation of this book to fill the gap. Consequently, user monitoring technology is considered a promising field, especially in long-term care. Advancing the monitoring of users of smart assisted technologies requires further studies to evaluate and demonstrate how they contribute to prolonging independent living. It is hoped that this book can facilitate this process.

As part of the book, a theory and practical issues and choices is presented, alongside a discussion of possible application contexts, technologies, and methodologies for processing data and modeling events using contemporary machine learning technologies. Extensive discussion focuses on how recent technological developments and changes in people's habits, due to advanced sensors in everyday life, will yield a vast amount of data. A critical aspect is the proper use of both technologies and data for healthy purposes. Unlike younger generations, elderly individuals may find it challenging and uninteresting to incorporate sensors, computers, or new technologies into their daily activities. Developing assisted living systems suitable for human–technology interactions, communication, and use requires considering psychosocial factors. These factors, along with data usage and processing, will likely necessitate further investigation by the scientific community to develop more sophisticated intelligent systems for care services, remote consultation, independent living support, social participation, well-being, and health condition monitoring.

ACKNOWLEDGEMENT

This chapter is partly supported by SMart Inclusive Living Environments (SMILE) project by European Union's Horizon 2020 Research and Innovation program, under Grant Agreement No. 101016848.

REFERENCES

[1] R. Z. Ur Rehman, C. Buckley, M. E. Micó-Amigo, C. Kirk, M. Dunne-Willows, C. Mazzá, J. Qing Shi, L. Alcock, L. Rochester, and S. Del Din, "Accelerometry-Based Digital Gait Characteristics for Classification of Parkinson's Disease: What Counts?" *IEEE Open Journal of Engineering in Medicine and Biology*, vol. 1, pp. 65–73, 2020.

[2] R. Lutze, "Practicality of Smartwatch Apps for Supporting Elderly People—A Comprehensive Survey," in: *Proceedings of the IEEE International Conference on Engineering, Technology and Innovation (ICE/ITMC)*; Stuttgart, Germany, June 2018, pp. 17–20.

[3] M. Haghi, A. Geissler, H. Fleischer, N. Stoll, and K. Thurow, "Ubiqsense: A Personal Wearable in Ambient Parameters Monitoring Based on IoT Platform," in: *Proceedings of the International Conference on Sensing and Instrumentation in IoT Era (ISSI)*; Lisbon, Portugal, August 29–30 2019.

[4] G. Paolini, D. Masotti, F. Antoniazzi, T. S. Cinotti, and A. Costanzo, "Fall Detection and 3-D Indoor Localization by a Custom RFID Reader Embedded in a Smart e-Health Platform," *IEEE Transactions on Microwave Theory and Techniques*, vol. 67, pp. 5329–5339, 2019.

[5] D. Ozgit, T. Butler, P. W. Oluwasanya, L. G. Occhipinti, and P. Hiralal, "Wear and Forget" Patch for Ambient Assisted Living," in: *Proceedings of the IEEE International Conference on Flexible and Printable Sensors and Systems (FLEPS)*; Glasgow, UK, July 8–10 2019.

[6] D. Rajamohanan, B. Hariharan, and K. A. Unnikrishna Menon, "Survey on Smart Health Management Using BLE and BLE Beacons," in: *Proceedings of the 9th International Symposium on Embedded Computing and System Design (ISED)*; Kollam, India, December 13–14 2019.

[7] D. Zambrano-Montenegro, R. García-Bermúdez, F. J. Bellido-Outeirino, J. M. Flores-Arias, and A. Huhn, "An Approach to Beacons-Based Location for AAL Systems in Broadband Communication Constrained Scenarios," in: *Proceedings of the IEEE 8th International Conference on Consumer Electronics—Berlin (ICCE-Berlin)*; Berlin, Germany, September 2–5 2018

[8] L. Ciabattoni, G. Foresi, A. Monteriù, L. Pepa; D. P. Pagnotta, L. Spalazzi, and F. Verdini, "Real Time Indoor Localization Integrating a Model Based Pedestrian Dead Reckoning on Smartphone and BLE Beacons," *Journal of Ambient Intelligence and Humanized Computing*, vol. 10, pp. 1–12, 2019.

[9] T. Morita, K. Taki, M. Fujimoto, H. Suwa, Y. Arakawa, and K. Yasumoto, "BLE Beacon-Based Activity Monitoring System toward Automatic Generation of Daily Report," in: *Proceedings of the IEEE International Conference on Pervasive Computing and Communications (PerCom 2018)*; Athens, Greece, March 19–23 2018.

[10] F. Cocconcelli, N. Mora, G. Matrella, P. Ciampolini "Seismocardiography-based Detection of Heartbeats for Continuous Monitoring of Vital Signs," in: *Proceedings of the 11th Computer Science and Electronic Engineering (CEEC)*; Colchester, UK, September 18–20 2019.

[11] N. Mora, F. Cocconcelli, G. Matrella, and P. Ciampolini, "Fully Automated Annotation of Seismocardiogram for Noninvasive Vital Sign Measurements," *IEEE Transactions on Instrumentation and Measurement*, vol. 69, p. 1241–1250, 2020.

[12] E. De-La-Hoz-Franco, P. Ariza-Colpas, J. M. Quero, and M. Espinilla, "Sensor-based Datasets for Human Activity Recognition - A Systematic Review of Literature," *IEEE Access*, vol. 6, 2018, doi: 10.1109/access.2018.2873502.59192

[13] M. A. U. Z. Chowdhury, M. R. Uddin, and A. A. Noman, "Human Activity Recognition Using Accelerometer, Gyroscope and Magnetometer Sensors: Deep Neural Network Approaches," in: A. K. M. Masum, E. H. Bahadur, and A. Shan-A-Alahi, Eds., *Proceedings of the 2019 10th International Conference on Computing*, Communication and Networking Technologies (ICCCNT); Kanpur, India, July 2019.

[14] M. Z. Uddin and A. Soylu, "Human Activity Recognition using Wearable Sensors, Discriminant Analysis, and Long Short-term Memory-based Neural Structured Learning," *Scientific Reports*, vol. 11, p. 16455, 2021, doi: 10.1038/s41598-021-95947-y

[15] W. Ugulino, D. Cardador, K. Vega, E. Velloso, R. Milidiu, and H. Fuks, "Wearable Computing: Accelerometers' Data Classification of Body Postures and Movements," in: *Proceedings of 21st Brazilian Symposium on Artificial Intelligence. Advances in Artificial Intelligence - SBIA 2012*, Lecture Notes in Computer Science, Curitiba, PR: Springer Berlin / Heidelberg, 2012, pp. 52–61. ISBN 978-3-642-34458-9, doi: 10.1007/978-3-642-34459-6_6

[16] F. Palumbo, C. Gallicchio, R. Pucci, and A. Micheli, "Human Activity Recognition Using Multisensor Data Fusion Based on Reservoir Computing," *Journal of Ambient Intelligence and Smart Environments*, vol. 8, no. 2, pp. 87–107, 2016.

[17] R. Sharma and R. B. Pachori, "Classification of Epileptic Seizures in EEG Signals Based on Phase Space Representation of Intrinsic Mode Functions," *Expert Systems with Applications*, vol. 42, no. 3, pp. 1106–1117, 2015, doi: 10.1016/j.eswa.2014.08.030

[18] J. R. Kwapisz, G. M. Weiss, and S. A. Moore, "Activity Recognition Using Cell Phone Accelerometers," *ACM SigKDD Explorations Newsletter*, vol. 12, no. 2, pp. 74–82, 2011, doi: 10.1145/1964897.1964918

[19] N. Y. Hammerla, S. Halloran, and T. Plötz, "Deep, Convolutional, and Recurrent Models for Human Activity Recognition Using Wearables," in: *Proceedings of the Twenty-Fifth International Joint Conference on Artificial Intelligence (IJCAI)*; New York, USA, 2016.

[20] M. Han Selmann, R. Stiefelhagen, and R. Dürichen, "CNN-Based Sensor Fusion Techniques for Multimodal Human Activity Recognition," in: S. Münzner, P. Schmidt, and A. Reiss, Eds., *Proceedings of the 2017 ACM International Symposium on Wearable Computers*; Maui, HI, USA, 2017, pp. 158–165.

[21] J.-L. Reyes-Ortiz, L. Oneto, A. Samà, X. Parra, and D. Anguita, "Transition-aware Human Activity Recognition Using Smartphones," *Neurocomputing*, vol. 171, pp. 754–767, 2016, doi: 10.1016/j.neucom.2015.07.085

[22] P. Siirtola, H. Koskimäki, and J. Röning, Eds, "Personal Models for eHealth-improving User-dependent Human Activity Recognition Models Using Noise Injection M," in: *Proceedings of the 2016 IEEE Symposium Series on Computational Intelligence (SSCI)*; Athens, Greece, December 2016.

[23] M. Botros, T. Heskes, and I. A. P. D. Vries, *Supervised Learning in Human Activity Recognition Based on Multimodal Body Sensing*, Doctoral dissertation, Radboud University, 2017.

[24] K. H. Walse, R. V. Dharaskar, and V. M. Thakare, "A Study of Human Activity Recognition Using AdaBoost Classifiers on WISDM Dataset," *The Institute of Integrative Omics and Applied Biotechnology Journal*, vol. 7, no. 2, pp. 68–76, 2016.

[25] J. Zhu, R. San-Segundo, and J. M. Pardo, "Feature Extraction for Robust Physical Activity Recognition," *Human-Centric Computing and Information Sciences*, vol. 7, no. 1, p. 16, 2017, doi: 10.1186/s13673-017-0097-2

[26] G. Vavoulas, C. Chatzaki, C. Chatzaki, T. Malliotakis, M. Pediaditis, and M. Tsiknakis, "The Mobiact Dataset: Recognition of Activities of Daily Living Using Smartphones," in: *Proceedings of the International Conference on Information and Communication Technologies for Ageing Well and e-Health*; Porto, Portugal, April 2016, pp. 143–151.

[27] L. Gorelick, M. Blank, E. Shechtman, M. Irani, and R. Basri, "Actions as Space-time Shapes," *IEEE Transactions on Pattern Analysis and Machine Intelligence*, vol. 29, no. 12, pp. 2247–2253, 2007.

[28] M. Zia Uddin, "Human Activity Recognition Using Segmented Body Part and Body Joint Features with Hidden Markov Models," *Multimedia Tools and Applications*, 2016, doi:10.1007/s11042-016-3742-2

[29] C. Schuldt, I. Laptev, and B. Caputo, "Recognizing Human Actions: A Local SVM Approach," in: *Proceedings of the 17th International Conference on Pattern Recognition (ICPR'04)*, 2004, pp. 32–36.

[30] J. Wang, Z. Liu, Y. Wu and J. Yuan, "Mining Actionlet Ensemble for Action Recognition with Depth Cameras," in: *2012 IEEE Conference on Computer Vision and Pattern Recognition*, 2012, pp. 1290–1297, doi: 10.1109/CVPR.2012.6247813

[31] C. Li, Q. Huang, X. Li, et al., "Human Action Recognition Based on Multi-scale Feature Maps from Depth Video Sequences," *Multimedia Tools and Applications*, vol. 80, pp. 32111–32130, 2021, doi: 10.1007/s11042-021-11193-4

[32] C. Y. Ma, M. H. Chen, Z. Kira, and G. AlRegib "TS-LSTM and Temporal-inception: Exploiting Spatiotemporal Dynamics for Activity Recognition. *Signal Processing: Image Communication*, vol. 71, pp. 76–87, 2019.

[33] A. Ahmed, A. Jalal, and K. Kim, "RGB-D Images for Object Segmentation, Localization and Recognition in Indoor Scenes Using Feature Descriptor and Hough Voting," in: *Proceedings of the 2020 17th International Bhurban Conference on Applied Sciences and Technology (IBCAST)*; Islamabad, Pakistan, January 14–18 2020, pp. 290–295.

[34] W. Sousa Lima, E. Souto, K. El-Khatib, R. Jalali, and J. Gama, "Human Activity Recognition Using Inertial Sensors in a Smartphone: An Overview," *Sensors*, vol. 19, p. 3213, 2019.

[35] J. Guo, Y. Li, M. Hou, S. Han, and J. Ren, "Recognition of Daily Activities of Two Residents in a Smart Home Based on Time Clustering," *Sensors*, vol. 20, p. 1457, 2020.

[36] Y. Liu, "OpenPose-Based Yoga Pose Classification Using Convolutional Neural Network," *Highlights in Science, Engineering and Technology*, vol. 23, pp. 72–76, 2022, doi: 10.54097/hset. v23i.3130

[37] J. L. Reyes-Ortiz, L. Oneto, A. Samà, X. Parra, D. Anguita, "Transition-Aware Human Activity Recognition Using Smartphones," *Neurocomputing*, vol. 171, pp. 754–767, 2016.

[38] L. Wang, Y. Xiong, Z. Wang, Y. Qiao, D. Lin, X. Tang, and L. Van Gool, "Temporal Segment Networks: Towards Good Practices for Deep Action Recognition," in: *European Conference on Computer Vision (ECCV)*; Springer: Amsterdam, The Netherlands, 2016, pp. 20–36.

[39] P. Wang, W. Li, Z. Gao, Y. Zhang, C. Tang, and P. Ogunbona, "Scene Flow to Action Map: A New Representation for RGB-D Based Action Recognition with Convolutional Neural Networks," in: *Proceedings of the IEEE Conference on Computer Vision and Pattern Recognition*, Honolulu, HI, USA, 21–26 July 2017.

[40] A. Gumaei, M. M. Hassan, A. Alelaiwi, and H. Alsalman, "A Hybrid Deep Learning Model for Human Activity Recognition Using Multimodal Body Sensing Data," *IEEE Access*, vol. 7, pp. 99152–99160, 2019.

[41] Y. Du, Y. Lim, Y. Tan, "A Novel Human Activity Recognition and Prediction in Smart Home Based on Interaction," *Sensors*, vol. 19, p. 4474, 2019.

[42] D. Bacciu, M. Di Rocco, M. Dragone, C. Gallicchio, A. Micheli, and A. Saffiotti, "An Ambient Intelligence Approach for Learning in Smart Robotic Environments," *Computational Intelligence*, vol. 35, pp. 1060–1087, 2019.

[43] S. Herath, M. Harandi, and F. Porikli Going Deeper Into Action Recognition: A Survey. *Image and Vision Computing*, 2017, 60, 4–21.

[44] H. W. Guesgen, "Using Rough Sets to Improve Activity Recognition Based on Sensor Data," *Sensors*, vol. 20, p. 1779, 2020.

[45] S. B. Uddin Tahir, A. Jalal, and M. Batool, "Wearable Sensors for Activity Analysis Using SMO-Based Random Forest over Smart Home and Sports Datasets," in: *Proceedings of the 2020 3rd International Conference on Advancements in Computational Sciences (ICACS)*; Lahore, Pakistan, February 17–19 2020, pp. 1–6.

[46] M. Shirali, M. Norouzi, M. Ghassemian, and D. Jai-Persad, "A Testbed Evaluation for an Indoor Temperature Monitoring System in Smart Homes," in: *Proceedings of the IEEE 20th International Conference on High Performance Computing and Communications*; Exeter, UK, June 28–30 2018.

[47] A. Veiga, L. García, L. Parra, J. Lloret, and V. Augele, "An IoT-based Smart Pillow for Sleep Quality Monitoring in AAL Environments," in: *Proceedings of the Third International Conference on Fog and Mobile Edge Computing (FMEC)*; Barcelona, Spain, April 23–26 2018.

[48] A.L. Bleda-Tomas, R. Maestre-Ferriz, M.Á. Beteta-Medina, J.A. Vidal-Poveda, "AmICare: Ambient Intelligent and Assistive System for Caregivers support," in: *Proceedings of the IEEE 16th International Conference on Embedded and Ubiquitous Computing (EUC)*; Bucharest, Romania, October 29–31 2018.

[49] M. P. Fanti, G. Faraut, J. J. Lesage, and M. Roccotelli, "An Integrated Framework for Binary Sensor Placement and Inhabitants Location Tracking," *IEEE Transactions on Systems, Man, and Cybernetics: Systems*, vol. 48, pp. 154–160, 2018.

[50] P. De, A. Chatterjee, and A. Rakshit, "PIR Sensor based AAL Tool for Human Movement Detection: Modified MCP based Dictionary Learning Approach," *IEEE Transactions on Instrumentation and Measurement*, vol. 69, pp. 7377–7385, 2020.

[51] A. R. Jimenez, F. Seco, P. Peltola, and M. Espinilla, "Location of Persons Using Binary Sensors and BLE Beacons for Ambient Assitive Living," in: *Proceedings of the 2018 International Conference on Indoor Positioning and Indoor Navigation (IPIN)*; Nantes, France, September 24–27 2018.

[52] S. Chen, "Toward Ambient Assistance: A Spatially Aware Virtual Assistant eNabled by Object Detection," in: *Proceedings of the International Conference on Computer Engineering and Application (ICCEA)*; Guangzhou, China, March 18–20 2020.

[53] S. Yue, Y. Yang, H. Wang, H. Rahul, and D. Katabi, "BodyCompass: Monitoring Sleep Posture with Wireless Signals," *Proceedings of the ACM on Interactive, Mobile, Wearable and Ubiquitous Technologies*, vol. 4, pp. 1–25, 2020.

[54] L. Fan, T. Li, Y. Yuan, and D. Katabi, "In-Home Daily-Life Captioning Using Radio Signals," *Computer Science—ECCV*, arXiv 2020, arXiv:2008.10966.

[55] Vahia, V.; Kabelac, Z.; YuHsu, C.; Forester, B.; Monette, P.; May, R.; Hobbs, K.; Munir, U.; Hoti, K.; Katabi, D. Radio Signal Sensing and Signal Processing to Monitor Behavioral Symptoms in Dementia: A Case Study. *The American Journal of Geriatric Psychiatry* 2020, 28, 820–825.

[56] L. Li, Y. Shuang, Q. Ma, H. Li, H. Zhao, M. L. Wei, C. Liu, C. Hao, C. Qiu, and T. Cui, "Intelligent Metasurface Imager and Recognizer," *Light: Science & Applications*, vol. 8, p. 97, 2019.

[57] Del Hougne, P.; Imani, M.; Diebold, A.; Horstmeyer, R.; Smith, D. Learned Integrated Sensing Pipeline: Reconfigurable Metasurface Transceivers as Trainable Physical Layer in an Artificial Neural Network. *Advanced Science*, vol. 7, p. 1901913, 2020.

[58] H. Y. Li, H. T. Zhao, M. L. Wei, H. X. Ruan, Y. Shuang, T. J. Cui, P. del Hougne, and L. Li, "Intelligent Electromagnetic Sensing with Learnable Data Acquisition and Processing," *Patterns*, vol. 1, p. 100006, 2020.

[59] I. Cebanov, C. Dobre, A. Gradinar, R. I. Ciobanu, and V. D. Stanciu, "Activity Recognition for Ambient Assisted Living Using Off – The Shelf Motion Sensing Input Devices," in: *Proceedings of the Global IoT Summit (GIoTS)*; Aarhus, Denmark, June 17–21 2019.

[60] K. Ryselis, T. Petkus, T. Blazauskas, R. Maskeliunas, and R. Damasevicius, "Multiple Kinect Based System to Monitor and Analyze Key Performance Indicators of Physical Training," *Human-centric Computing and Information Sciences*, vol. 10, p. 51, 2020.

[61] D. J. Cook, A. S. Crandall, B. L. Thomas, and N. C. Krishnan, "CASAS: A Smart Home in a Box," *Computer*, vol. 46, no. 7, pp. 62–69, 2013.

[62] D. Liciotti, M. Bernardini, L. Romeo, and E. Frontoni, "A Sequential Deep Learning Application for Recognising Human Activities in Smart Homes," *Neurocomputing*, vol. 396, pp. 501–513, 2020.

[63] Develco Products. Available: https://www.develcoproducts.com. [Accessed: 04/02/2024].

[64] N. Gürsakal, S. Çelik, and E. Birişçi, "Synthetic Data Generation with Python," *Synthetic Data for Deep Learning*, vol. 1, pp. 159–214, 2022, doi: 10.1007/978-1-4842-8587-9_5

[65] S. Tsimfer, "ML-Aware Synthetic Data Generation," in: *Second EAGE Subsurface Intelligence Workshop*, 2022, doi: 10.3997/2214-4609.2022616024

## CHAPTER 6

Emotion Recognition

6.1 IMAGE-BASED EMOTION RECOGNITION

Image-based emotion recognition aims to help computers understand human emotions by analyzing facial expressions in pictures. This process mimics how we naturally interpret emotions by looking at subtle signals in people's faces, like a smile for joy, a furrowed brow for concern, or widened eyes for surprise. These details serve as the foundation for training machines to understand and respond to human emotions. Image-based emotion recognition typically starts by identifying faces in images [1–29]. After finding a face, the computer focuses on specific facial features like eyes, nose, and mouth, using them as reference points to analyze the structure and movement of facial expressions. Deep learning, a vital part of AI, takes a central role in image-based emotion recognition, with Convolutional Neural Networks (CNNs) being essential tools. These models undergo extensive training on various datasets containing images displaying diverse emotional expressions. Through this training, the computer learns to recognize patterns and features associated with different emotions, forming the basis for subsequent recognition. Techniques like facial landmark detection and CNNs are crucial in unraveling the complexities of facial images, enabling the computer to learn and distinguish subtle variations in expressions and enhancing its ability to recognize and categorize emotions accurately.

However, this technological journey comes with challenges, such as variability in facial expressions, cultural differences, and inconsistent accuracy. Robust algorithms are essential to navigate this complex web of variations, ensuring the reliability and applicability of image-based emotion recognition in diverse situations. The significance of image-based emotion recognition extends beyond theories, finding practical applications in various domains. In human–computer interaction, envision a computer not only perceiving your joy but responding with a cheerful message or adjusting its behavior to match your mood. This transformative potential highlights this technology's profound impact of image-based emotion recognition can be integrated. By assessing students' engagement and emotional states during online classes, educators can customize to suit the emotional dynamics of their students for better performance. Adapting and responding to the learning environment's emotional

DOI: 10.1201/9781003425908-6

context holds promise in creating more effective and engaging educational experiences. In healthcare, image-based emotion recognition emerges as a potential tool for assessing mental health. Healthcare professionals can gain valuable insights into patients' emotional well-being by analyzing facial expressions, providing a nuanced understanding beyond traditional diagnostic methods. The potential for early detection and intervention in conditions like depression and anxiety holds significant promise for improving mental health outcomes.

Despite these applications, challenges persist, prompting a critical examination of the technology's limitations. Variability in facial expressions, cultural nuances, and ethical considerations related to privacy and potential biases in recognition systems require careful consideration. The responsible deployment of image-based emotion recognition technology demands a delicate balance between innovation and ethical considerations.

Facial expression recognition serves as the most intuitive way to convey human emotions. Over recent decades, significant research efforts have been directed toward recognizing facial expressions from videos [1, 2]. A standard expression recognition system involves acquiring face images, extracting features, training, and recognition. Most facial image features are highly sensitive to noise and variations in illumination. Therefore, features capable of tolerating noise and changes in illumination play a crucial role in constructing a resilient expression recognition system. Figure 6.1 illustrates the basic flowchart of vision-based facial expression recognition, where the training part explains how to train a model later used in the testing part.

In the process of extracting facial expression features from images, Principal Component Analysis (PCA) has been widely used [3–6]. PCA was applied in [3] to understand facial expression images. In [5, 6], PCA played a role in facial adapting and responding to the learning environment's emotional context action coding system for expression recognition. Researchers have explored Independent Component Analysis (ICA), a statistical approach higher in order than PCA, for face and facial expression analysis [5, 10–21]. In [14], ICA features were combined with support vectors to depict various facial expressions. Figure 6.2 displays some sample faces, while Figure 6.3 showcases PCA and ICA basis images, with PCA representing global features and ICA capturing local features.

Local Binary Patterns (LBP) have been used in some research for facial expression analysis [22–26]. LBP is notable for its resilience against variations in illumination. It underwent refinement, evolving into Local Directional Pattern (LDP) [25], which focuses on a pixel's gradient information to portray local features [2, 25, 26]. LDP features exhibit superior tolerance compared to LBP in handling illumination variation in image sequences as they concentrate on a pixel's gradient information [25]. The empirical determination of the number of top strength directions characterizes LDP.

Hidden Markov Models (HMM) have been widely adopted in various research works to train and recognize facial expressions from depth and RGB videos. Recently, the attention of artificial intelligence and machine learning researchers has shifted toward deep learning methods [30–32]. The initial deep learning technique was the Deep Belief Network (DBN) using Restricted Boltzmann Machines (RBMs). The incorporation of RBM makes DBN training notably faster than DNN. Additionally, Convolutional Neural Networks (CNN)

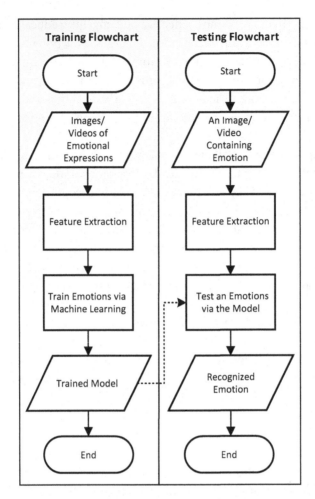

FIGURE 6.1   Basic flowchart of machine learning-based emotion recognition from images/videos.

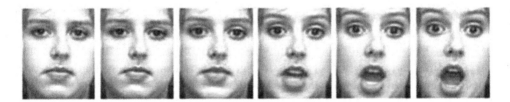

FIGURE 6.2   A sequential facial expression images of surprise.

have gained popularity due to its enhanced discriminative power compared to DNN and DBN. Essentially, CNN, a form of deep learning, involves feature extractions alongside convolutional stacks, forming a progressive hierarchy of abstract features. The constituent elements of a CNN encompass convolution, pooling, tangent squashing, rectifier, and normalization. CNN adopts a hierarchical structure where convolutional layers alternate with subsampling layers, culminating in a fully connected layer. The fully connected layer mirrors a conventional multilayer perceptron-based neural network. CNN-based deep

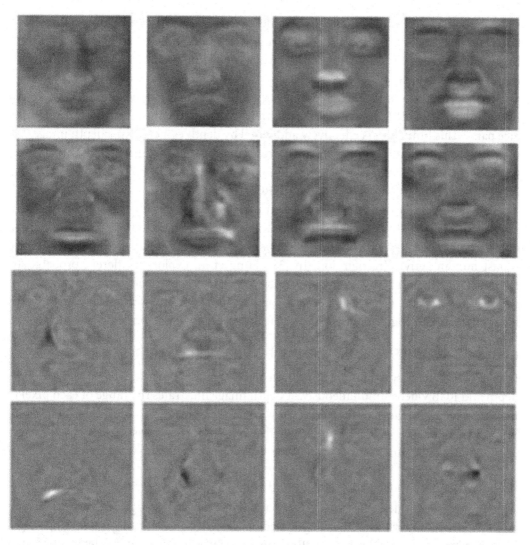

FIGURE 6.3   Eight basis images after applying PCA (top) and ICA (bottom) on the facial expression images of the six expressions: namely anger, joy, sad, disgust, fear, and surprise.

learning primarily finds application in efficiently recognizing patterns in a visual scene, such as object detection in extensive image datasets. With appropriate training, the convolutional layers of a CNN can discern salient features, and the fully connected layer can generate final classification vectors. In scenarios with limited training data, CNNs demonstrate superior classification performance in contrast to intricate models used for typical deep learning tasks. Consequently, simple 1-D CNNs prove easier to train within fewer epochs than conventional 2-D CNNs [30]. Hence, 1-D CNN facilitates rapid classification of facial expressions utilizing features from a restricted number of facial expression videos. Given CNN's suitability for deep learning-based pattern analysis, it emerges as an apt candidate to model and decode facial features in expression recognition systems. Several researchers have scrutinized deep learning approaches for expression recognition based on static RGB images [33–36]. Despite the prevalent use of static images in expression recognition research, videos offer a more comprehensive representation of emotional information [2, 26]. Therefore, videos constitute appropriate inputs for a resilient expression recognition system.

For capturing face images, RGB cameras are the most employed devices [33–36]. An inherent limitation of RGB cameras lies in the absence of depth information for distinct face parts. This limitation is effectively addressed by depth cameras. In a depth image, the intensity distribution of a face pixel corresponds to the distance from the camera. Consequently, depth images emerge as superior representations of face components (e.g., nose, eyebrows, lips) compared to standard RGB images for expression recognition. Depth cameras have found extensive application in various computer vision and image processing domains [37–39]. In [37], surface histograms on depth images were analyzed for human activity recognition. [38] involved the analysis of moving body parts from depth data for robust human activity recognition. In [39], Sung et al. explored different probabilistic approaches to human activities in depth and color videos. Depth videos prove valuable for establishing a robust facial expression recognition system. This section has investigated facial expression recognition using diverse features and machine learning algorithms.

6.2 CASE STUDIES FOR IMAGE-BASED EMOTION RECOGNITION

Images of various expressions are taken by a depth camera [2]. The depth camera produces depth and RGB videos simultaneously. A depth image illustrates the range of each pixel in the scene; longer-range pixels are depicted with dark values, and shorter-range pixels with bright values. Figure 6.4 displays a sample depth image of a surprise expression (top left), corresponding grey (top right), depth (bottom left), and pseudo image (bottom right).

6.2.1 Local Directional Strength Pattern (LDSP)

Among several edge detectors for a pixel in an image, the Kirsch edge detector [25] detects edges more accurately than other edge detectors since it considers all surrounding neighbors. The local directional ranks (LDRs) T to a specific direction can be determined after applying the Kirsch masks s as

$$T_D = \sum_{x,y} R\{s(x,y) = v\}, v = (1,...8),$$

$$\text{Direction} \in E, SE, S, SW, W, NW, N, NE,$$

For a pixel, edge response values are calculated using the Kirsch masks [26] in eight different orientations centered on its position, as shown in Figures 6.5 and 6.6 shows results of applying eight Kirsch edge masks on a depth face.

As can be noticed there, each direction represents the edge responses. Hence, generating a pattern considering all directions should produce robust features. Figure 6.7 shows directional responses for a central pixel and ranking of the directions based on edge strengths. The Local Directional Strength Pattern (LDSP) assigns an eight-bit binary code to each pixel of a depth face. This pattern is calculated by considering positions with highest edge

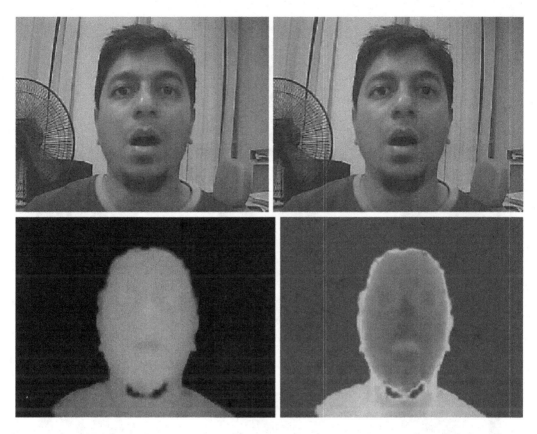

FIGURE 6.4   (a) An RGB, (b) corresponding gray, (c) depth, and (d) pseudo image of a surprise expression.

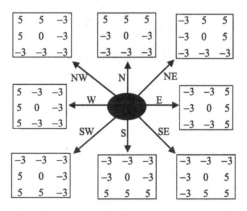

FIGURE 6.5   Kirsch edge masks in eight surrounding directions.

strengths in bright and dark regions for a pixel. For a pixel in the image, the eight directional edge response values are calculated by Kirsch masks. In typical LDP, absolute values of edge responses are taken. Then, directions representing top absolute strengths are set to 1 and rest of them 0. Unlike LDP, the strengths are kept with their signs. Then, the binary positions with highest and lowest strength values are considered.

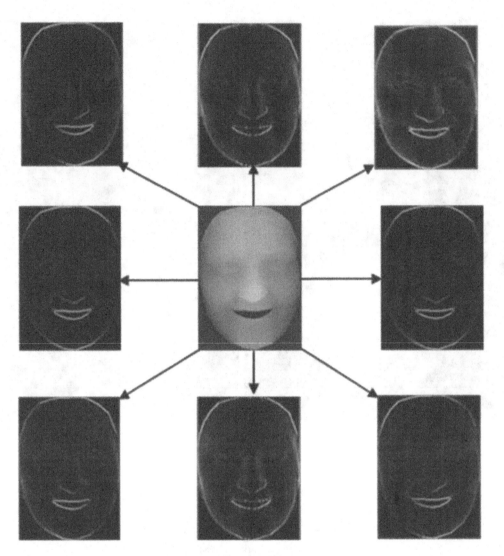

FIGURE 6.6   Edge response to eight directions for a depth face.

S_{NW}	S_N	S_{NE}
S_W	X	S_E
S_{SW}	S_S	S_{SE}

(a)

R_{NW}	R_N	R_{NE}
R_W	X	R_E
R_{SW}	R_S	R_{SE}

(b)

FIGURE 6.7   (a) Edge response to eight directions and (b) ranking of the directions based on edge strengths.

LDSP patterns represent robust features for salient pixels in an image, especially edge pixels. Thus, the LDSP code for a pixel x is derived as

$$\text{LDSP}(x) = \sum_{i=0}^{5} (D_i \times 2^i),$$

$$D = \text{binary}\big(\arg(s(h))\big) \big\| \text{binary}\big(\arg(s(l))\big),$$

$$\text{binary}(f) = \big((\lfloor f/4 \rfloor)\%2\big) \big\| \big((\lfloor f/2 \rfloor)\%2\big) \big\| (f\%2)$$

where h represents the highest edge response direction and l the lowest edge response direction. Figure 6.8 shows two examples of LDSP codes where typical LDP makes the *same* patterns for different edges but LDSP can generate *separate* patterns. In the upper part of the figure, the highest edge response is 1452. Hence, the first three bits of the LDSP code is the binary representation of the direction 4 i.e., 100. The highest edge response in the dark side is −2108 and hence the last three bits of the LDSP are the binary of the direction 1 i.e., 001. Hence, the LDSP code for the upper pixel is 100001. Similarly, the LDSP code for the lower pixel is 001100, a separate pattern to the upper pixel. On the other hand, LDP codes for both are the same, considering all possible top strengths since the rankings in all the directions are exactly the same for both pixels. Hence, the LDSP code represents better features than LDP. Figure 6.9 shows a LDSP histogram for a sample depth face. Thus, an image is transformed to the LDSP histogram map using LDSP code where n^{th} bin can be defined as

$$P_n = \sum_{x,y} I\{LDSP(x,y) = n\}, n = (0,1,\ldots m-1)$$

where m is the number of the LDSP histogram bins. Then, the histogram of the LDSP map for a face region is presented as

$$\text{Histogram}_{(\text{LDSP})} = (P_0, P_1, \ldots, P_{m-1}).$$

where u represents the number of non-overlapped regions in the image.

6.2.2 Principal Component Analysis on LDSP

The next stage in the feature extraction procedure involves the application of Principal Component Analysis (PCA) on LDSP features. PCA is essentially a statistical method of lower order used to transform original high-dimensional data into a feature space of lower dimensions. The process begins by computing eigenvectors of the covariance data matrix, followed by an approximation of the linear combination of the top eigenvectors or principal components. PCA is widely employed in pattern analysis research to reduce the dimensionality of high-dimensional features. PCA is designed for linear structures which makes it effective in identifying directions with maximum variations. Thus, it faces challenges in characterizing data with nonlinear structures. Therefore, the feature vectors for a depth face using PCA can be expressed as.

$$K = ME_m^T.$$

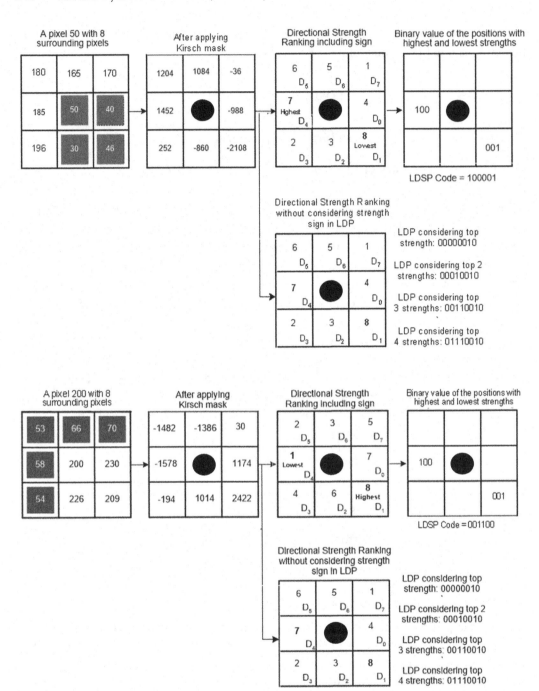

FIGURE 6.8   Two examples for different kind of edge pixels where LDP fails to separate them but LDSP separates them successfully.

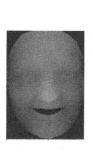
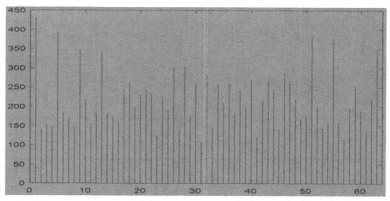

FIGURE 6.9   LDSP histogram for a sample depth face.

6.2.3 Linear Discriminant Analysis on PCA

In Linear Discriminant Analysis (LDA), the class separation criterion is typically determined by the ratio of between-class and within-class properties. LDA can be extended using Gaussian kernel functions, allowing the principal components in the transformed kernel space to establish nonlinear relationships with the input variables. Consequently, the objective of LDA is to maximize the following criterion as

$$\Lambda = \frac{\left|V^T Z_B V\right|}{\left|V^T Z_T V\right|}$$

where Z_B and Z_T are the between-class and within-class scatters matrices. Finally, the PCA features K of a face image is projected on LDA space $Z_{(LDA)}$ as

$$Q = Z_{(LDA)}^T K.$$

For every expression, there are 39 training videos, with each video containing 10 frames. This results in a total of 2340 samples across six different expressions in each plot.

6.2.4 Facial Expression Modeling

The spatiotemporal features extracted from depth videos undergo application in a Convolutional Neural Network (CNN) for the modeling of diverse facial expressions. CNN, primarily employed in image-based deep learning applications, often outperforms other deep learning structures in machine learning applications due to its proficiency in extracting and learning image-based features [32]. Additionally, CNN possesses the advantage of utilizing fewer bias and weight values compared to alternative deep learning methods.

Illustrated in Figure 6.10 is the configuration of the 1-D CNN employed in this study. LDA features derived from an expression video comprising 10 frames are structured as 10 × 150 and serve as inputs to the CNN. The network comprises three convolution layers, three pooling layers, and one fully connected layer. The network's output is categorized into normal

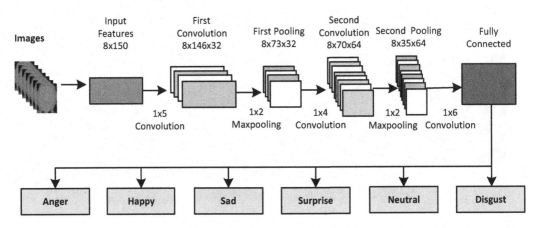

FIGURE 6.10   Basic architecture of the 1-D CNN used in this work.

and abnormal expressions through a fully connected layer. In the initial convolution layer, Convolution-1, the input matrix undergoes convolution with 32 kernels, each sized 1×5, resulting in a matrix of $10 \times 146 \times 32$.

$$\text{Convolution}_{k}^{(i+1)}(m,n) = ReLU(u),$$

$$ReLU((u)) = \sum_{(g=1)}^{z} \Omega\left(m, \left(n - g + \frac{z+1}{2}\right)\right) W_{k}^{i}(g) + \alpha_{k}^{i}$$

where $\text{Convolution}_{k}^{(i+1)}(m,n)$ generates convolution results for (m, n) coordinates of the $(i + 1)$th layer with kth convolution map. W_{k}^{i} is the kth *convolution kernel* for the ith layer. α_{k}^{i} is the kth *bias values* for the ith layer. Ω is the map of the previous layer and z the size of the kernel. *ReLU* represents the active function that considers the summation of weights of the previous layer to pass them to the next layer. The second layer is the first pooling layer *Pooling₁*. This layer basically down samples the results of *Convolution₁* to a matrix of $8 \times 73 \times 32$ via 1×2 max pooling. In pooling, the maximum value is selected from applying a 1×2 sliding window in the output of previous convolutional layer.

Thus, the pooling results for $(i + 1)$th layer, kernel k, row x, and column y can be represented as

$$\text{Pooling}_{k}^{i+1}(x, y) = \max_{1 \le r \le s}\left(\text{Convolution}_{k}^{i}\left(x, \left((y-1)*r + s\right)\right)\right)$$

where p is the length of the pooling window. Using a similar way, the second convolution layer applies 64 convolution kernels with the size of 1×4. Similar to the first pooling layer, 1×2 max-pooling is applied for second pooling layer. At last, the fully connected layer is obtained as

$$FC_{j}^{(l+1)} = ReLU\left(\sum_{i} x_{i}^{l} W_{ij}^{l} + \alpha_{j}^{l}\right)$$

where W_{ij}^l is a matrix containing weight values from the ith node of the lth layer to the jth node of the $(l+1)$th layer. x_i^l represents the content of ith node at lth layer.

6.2.5 Experiments on Depth Dataset

For the experiments, a facial expression database based on depth videos was recorded. This database included RGB and depth videos capturing frontal faces expressing six different emotions: surprise, sad, happy, disgust, anger, and neutral. The videos assumed minimal head motion, which was neglected during the recordings. There were 40 videos for each expression. The experimental setup involved leave-one-out cross-validation, or 40-fold cross-validation, on the videos corresponding to each facial expression. In each fold, 39 videos were utilized for training, and one video was reserved for testing. The results from these 40 folds were aggregated to determine the final recognition rate.

For training and testing, a total of 1560 videos were used for each facial expression, with 40 videos allocated for testing. Figure 6.11 displays sample depth faces depicting happy and surprise expressions from the database. The experimental setups for depth camera-based experiments mirrored those for RGB camera-based ones. The average recognition rates using ICA and HMM on depth faces reached 84.58%, as detailed in Table 6.1. Employing LDP with HMM on depth facial expression images resulted in an average recognition rate of 88.33%. LD2BP with HMM achieved a higher average recognition rate at 89.58%. Further, applying LDPP-LDA features with DBN yielded a commendable average recognition rate of 92.91%. Finally, the proposed architecture (i.e., LDSP-PCA-LDA with CNN) outperformed others, attaining the highest average recognition rate at 97.08%. This underscores the superiority of the proposed approach. Figure 6.12 illustrates the recognition

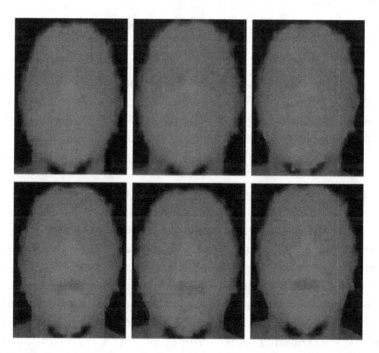

FIGURE 6.11   Sample depth faces of happy and surprise expressions from a depth database.

TABLE 6.1   Results Using Different Approaches from a Depth Database

	Anger	Happy	Sad	Neutral	Surprise	Disgust	Average
ICA-HMM (RGB)	77.5	85	82.5	80	82.5	82.5	**81.66**
LDP-HMM (RGB)	85	80	80	85	82.5	80	**82.08**
LD2BP -HMM (RGB)	85	82.5	82.5	87.5	85	82.5	**84.16**
LDPP-LDA-DBN (RGB)	90	90	87.5	92.5	92.5	90	**90.41**
LDSP-PCA-LDA-DBN (RGB)	92.5	95	92.5	95	95	92.5	**93.75**
ICA-HMM (Depth)	82.5	85	85	87.5	85	82.5	**84.58**
LDP-HMM (Depth)	90	87.5	87.5	90	90	85	**88.33**
LD2BP -HMM (Depth)	90	87.5	90	92.5	90	87.5	**89.58**
LDPP-LDA-DBN (Depth)	92.5	90	90	97.5	95	92.5	**92.91**
LDSP-PCA-LDA-CNN (Depth)	97.5	97.5	95	97.5	97.5	97.5	**97.08**

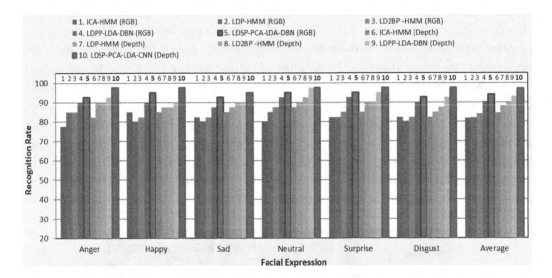

FIGURE 6.12   Sample depth faces of happy and surprise expressions from a depth database.

rates of various approaches based on both RGB and depth faces, with the proposed method exhibiting the highest recognition rate.

6.2.6 Experiments on RGB-based Public Database

Various approaches on the Cohn-Kanade facial expression database [40] have been tried to evaluate the resilience of LDSP-PCA-LDA features with CNN. This database, an extended version of [41], encompasses six facial expressions captured by RGB cameras from 123 subjects: anger, happy, sadness, surprise, fear, and disgust. Sample images of happy and surprise expressions from the public database are presented in Figures 6.13. Each expression involved 40 videos from distinct subjects, and leave-one-out cross-validation was applied for training and testing expression classification. The results of different approaches on the dataset are tabulated in Table 6.2, with LDSP-PCA-LDA features combined with CNN exhibiting higher accuracy. For improved visualization, Figure 6.14 illustrates these results.

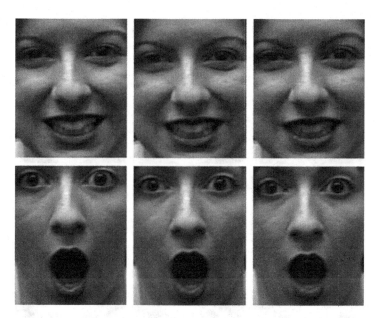

FIGURE 6.13   Sample grey faces of happy and surprise expressions from the Cohn-Kanade database.

TABLE 6.2   Results Using Different Approaches from CK Database

	Anger	Happy	Sad	Neutral	Surprise	Disgust	Average
ICA-HMM	55	60	82.5	77.5	57.5	75	**67.91**
LDP-HMM	67.5	75	85	87.5	62.5	75	**75.41**
LD2BP-HMM	82.5	82.5	87.5	90	87.5	85	**85.83**
LDPP-LDA-DBN	92.5	95	92.5	95	92.5	92.5	**93.33**
LDSP-PCA-LDA-CNN	95	97.5	97.5	97.5	95	95	**96.25**

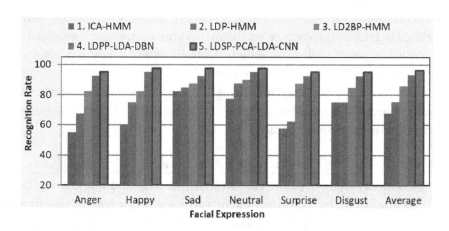

FIGURE 6.14   Results using different approaches on CK dataset.

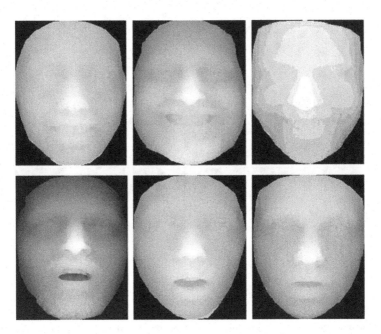

FIGURE 6.15 Some happy and surprise images from Bosphorus database.

TABLE 6.3 Results Using Different Approaches from Bosphorus Database

	Anger	Happy	Sad	Neutral	Surprise	Disgust	Average
ICA-HMM	55	62.5	85	80	65	67.5	69.16
LDP-HMM	52.5	60	87.5	82.5	67.5	70	70
LD2BP-HMM	90	87.5	90	95	90	87.5	90
LDPP-LDA-DBN	92.5	92.5	90	95	90	92.5	92.08
LDSP-PCA-LDA-CNN	95	97.5	92.5	97.5	95	95	95.41

6.2.7 Experiments on Depth-based Public Database

Various methodologies were applied to the Bosphorus public database, encompassing six 3-D facial expressions enacted by 105 subjects [42–44]. Utilizing depth information-based data, we aimed to train and recognize six distinct expressions: anger, happy, sad, surprise, fear, and disgust. Figure 6.15 displays sample depth images of happy and surprise expressions from the database. For each expression, sixty-five videos from different subjects were allocated for training, and 40 videos for testing. Table 6.3 presents the outcomes of diverse approaches on the publicly available depth dataset, with LDSP-PCA-LDA features coupled with CNN exhibiting superior accuracy.

6.3 SAMPLE CODE FOR IMAGE-BASED EMOTION RECOGNITION

Let's save the FER2013 dataset in the current folder as train and test folders. The images can be downloaded from the following link: https://www.kaggle.com/datasets/msambare/fer2013. The dataset is quite popular and should be available in many archives all over the Internet. Figure 6.16 shows the confusion matrix of seven universal facial expression

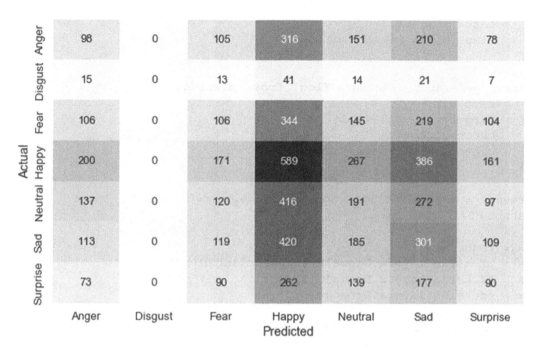

FIGURE 6.16   Confusion matrix of seven universal facial expression recognition using FER-2013 dataset and ResNet50.

recognition using FER-2013 dataset and ResNet50, according to the following source code. In the code, the training and testing folders are for saving the training and testing images to run the further experiment of deep learning.

```
import matplotlib.pyplot as plt
import tensorflow as tf
from tensorflow.keras.preprocessing.image import
ImageDataGenerator
from tensorflow.keras.optimizers import Adam
from tensorflow.keras.applications import ResNet50V2 as ResNet
from tensorflow.keras.callbacks import EarlyStopping

batch_size = 64

precision = tf.keras.metrics.Precision(name='precision')
recall = tf.keras.metrics.Recall(name='recall')
auc_roc = tf.keras.metrics.AUC(num_thresholds=200, name='auc_roc')
train_dir = "./train/"
test_dir = "./test"
num_classes = 7
datagen = ImageDataGenerator(rescale=1 / 255)

train_generator = datagen.flow_from_directory(
    train_dir,
    target_size=(224, 224),
```

```python
    batch_size=64,
    class_mode='categorical'
)

test_generator = datagen.flow_from_directory(
    test_dir,
    target_size=(224, 224),
    batch_size=64,
    class_mode='categorical'
)

resnet = ResNet(include_top=False, weights='imagenet', input_
shape=(224, 224, 3))

x = resnet.output
x = tf.keras.layers.GlobalAveragePooling2D()(x)
x = tf.keras.layers.Dense(512, activation='relu')(x)
x = tf.keras.layers.Dropout(0.5)(x)

predictions = tf.keras.layers.Dense(num_classes,
activation='softmax')(x)

model = tf.keras.models.Model(inputs=resnet.input,
outputs=predictions)
for layer in resnet.layers:
    layer.trainable = False

model.compile(optimizer=Adam(learning_rate=0.001),
            loss='categorical_crossentropy',
            metrics=['accuracy', precision, recall, auc_roc])

history = model.fit(train_generator,
            epochs=2,
            validation_data=test_generator)


plt.plot(history.history['loss'], label='train_loss')
plt.title('Training  Loss')
plt.xlabel('Epoch')
plt.ylabel('Loss')
plt.legend()
plt.show()

import numpy as np
preds = model.predict(test_generator)
y_preds = np.argmax(preds , axis = 1 )
y_test = np.array(test_generator.labels)

import pandas as pd
import seaborn as sns
from sklearn.metrics import confusion_matrix
```

```
Emotions = ['Anger', 'Disgust', 'Fear', 'Happy', 'Neutral',
'Sad', "Surprise"]
cm_data = confusion_matrix(y_test, y_preds)
cm = pd.DataFrame(cm_data, columns=Emotions, index = Emotions)
cm.index.name = 'Actual'
cm.columns.name = 'Predicted'
plt.figure(figsize = (20,10))
plt.title('Confusion Matrix', fontsize = 10)
sns.set(font_scale=1.2)
ax = sns.heatmap(cm, cbar=False, cmap="Blues", annot=True, annot_
kws={"size": 13}, fmt='g')
```

6.4 REAL-TIME IMAGE-BASED EMOTION RECOGNITION

We can use a library called deepface for real-time face detection and emotion recognition. Let's install deepface as *pip install deepface* and opencv as *pip install opencv-python*. A face cascade HAAR classifier file should be loaded in the same folder. The file is available in many links, one of them can be here https://raw.githubusercontent.com/opencv/opencv/master/data/haarcascades/haarcascade_frontalface_default.xml. Then execute the following code.

```
import cv2
from deepface import DeepFace
import os

os.environ['CUDA _ VISIBLE _ DEVICES'] = '-1'

# Load the pre-trained emotion detection model
Emo_model = DeepFace.build_model("Emotion")

# Define emotion categories
emotion_labels = ['angry', 'disgust', 'fear', 'happy', 'sad',
'surprise', 'neutral']

# Load face cascade HAAR classifier
face_HAAR_cascade = cv2.CascadeClassifier(cv2.data.haarcascades +
'haarcascade_frontalface_default.xml')

# Start Camera
Cap = cv2.VideoCapture(0)

while 1:
    # Capture frame
    ret, img = Cap.read()
    # Make frame to grayscale
    gray = cv2.cvtColor(img, cv2.COLOR_BGR2GRAY)

    # Face detection
    faces = face_HAAR_cascade.detectMultiScale(gray,
scaleFactor=1.1, minNeighbors=5, minSize=(30, 30))

    # Face coordinates
    for (x, y, w, h) in faces:
```

```
                # Extract the face from whole image
                face = gray[y:y + h, x:x + w]

                # Resize the face to match the input to deep model
                resized = cv2.resize(face, (48, 48), interpolation=cv2.
INTER_AREA)

                # Normalize face
                normalized = resized / 255.0

                # Reshape the image
                reshaped = normalized.reshape(1, 48, 48, 1)

                # Prediction of emotions using the pre-trained model
                pred = Emo_model.predict(reshaped)[0]
                id = pred.argmax()
                emotion = emotion_labels[id]

                # Draw rectangle around face and label with predicted emotion
                cv2.rectangle(img, (x, y), (x + w, y + h), (0, 0, 255), 2)
                cv2.putText(img, emotion, (x, y - 10), cv2.FONT_HERSHEY_
SIMPLEX, 0.9, (0, 0, 255), 2)

        # Show Frame with Emotion Categories
        cv2.imshow('Real-time Emotion Detection', img)

        # Press 'q' to exit
        if cv2.waitKey(1) & 0xFF == ord('e'):
            break

# Release the capture and close all windows
Cap.release()
cv2.destroyAllWindows()
```

Different real-time emotion detection results are shown as bellow in Figure 6.17.

Real-time facial expression recognition can be extended more with explainable artificial intelligence techniques such as the following archive. Figure 6.18 shows real-time facial expression recognition using ensemble learning and explanations.

https://github.com/siqueira-hc/Efficient-Facial-Feature-Learning-with-Wide-Ensemble-based-Convolutional-Neural-Networks

6.5 VOICE-BASED EMOTION RECOGNITION

Human–computer interaction (HCI) is gaining considerable attention from numerous researchers due to its practical applications in ubiquitous systems [44–80]. For instance, integrating HCI systems into a ubiquitous healthcare system can enhance the system by accurately perceiving people's emotions and proactively acting to improve their life-style. Research on emotion recognition from audio is garnering attention in HCI for emotional healthcare in smartly controlled environments [45]. Speech, a natural human

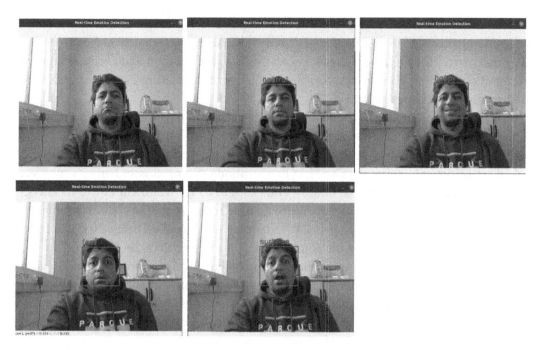

FIGURE 6.17   Results from real-time facial expression recognition.

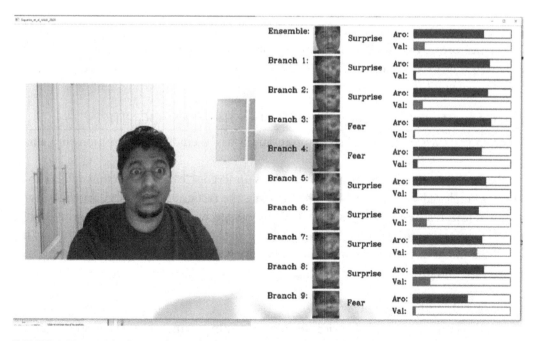

FIGURE 6.18   Results from real-time facial expression recognition and explanations.

communication method, plays a crucial role in affective computing research, contributing to the development of harmonious HCI systems, with emotion recognition from speech as a primary step. However, the lack of an exact definition of emotion makes robust emotion recognition from audio speech a complex challenge, necessitating extensive research to address the underlying problems [46].

Sound is a pressure wave resulting from the vibration of molecules in a substance. Sound waves, generated from a single source, typically propagate in all directions, exerting physical pressure on our ears. These waves are interpreted as electrical signals when transmitted to neurons [47–53]. When a sound wave originates from its source, it vibrates particles such as solids, liquids, and gases in its environment due to its energy. Sound waves always require a material form (solid, liquid, or gas) in the environment to travel. Sound waves can be categorized based on their frequencies: below 20 Hz, between 20 and 20000 Hz (human audible sound waves), and more than 20000 Hz (ultrasonic sound waves). Sound waves find applications in science and technology, such as ultrasound devices for imaging internal organs and breaking up kidney stones. Speech signals convey the feelings and intentions of the speaker, and signal analysis in both time and frequency domains can provide features to model underlying events, including speaker identification, speech, and emotion.

In the study of affective identification of speech information, the typical approach involves raw audio signal processing followed by learning extracted features with models like CNN and LSTM for comprehensive pattern recognition or event prediction. Spectrogram analysis of the speech signal, where the signal is windowed into small chunks and divided into narrowband and broadband spectrums, is common for speech pattern recognition [54]. Emotion recognition from the speech signal based on the spectrum can significantly contribute to the feature engineering process. In [55], authors studied spectrogram with CNN and SVM for emotion recognition. In [56], deep CNN was applied to extract features from the spectrogram of emotional speech. In [57], a two-dimensional spectrogram with CNN and LSTM was used for emotion recognition. This section explored voice-based emotion recognition.

6.6 CASE STUDIES ON VOICE-BASED EMOTION RECOGNITION

Figure 6.19 shows a schematic setup of an audio-based emotion recognition in a smart room.

The audio sensor data capturing all emotions undergoes feature extraction and is subsequently employed to train a NSL model. During the recognition process, an edge device acquires features from a small segment of audio speech and applies them to the trained model for emotion recognition. Figure 6.20 illustrates the fundamental architecture of the proposed method, encompassing signal data collection, feature extraction, training, and the recognition process.

6.6.1 Signal Pre-processing

A sound signal exists in an electrical form representing sound. Analog sound signals are identical copies of the sound, while digital sound signals are numerical representations

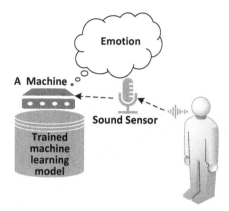

FIGURE 6.19 A schematic picture of audio-based emotion recognition for human machine interaction in a room.

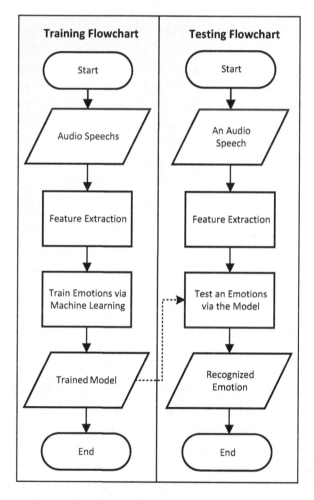

FIGURE 6.20 Training and testing flowcharts of the proposed system.

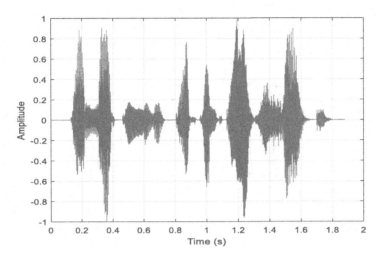

FIGURE 6.21   A sample anger audio file from the experimental dataset.

derived from analog sound through sampling and transformation into digital form, ranging between 1 and 0, as depicted in Figure 6.21. Speech signals are inherently complex signals with varying frequencies, analyzed using a spectrogram [60–79]. The Fast Fourier Transform (FFT) is the most widely used method for spectrogram analysis in such signals.

FFT is employed on a signal window to transform a sound signal from the time domain to the frequency domain. It serves as a measure of signal frequencies through spectrogram analysis, depicting the intensity of vibrations across different frequencies. FFT employs a fast algorithm to mitigate time complexity in computing the Discrete Fourier Transform (DFT). This transformation is performed to efficiently analyze the frequency components of the signal.

$$Q_k = \sum_{n=0}^{(N-1)} Q_n e^{-i*\left(\frac{2\pi kn}{N}\right)} \qquad k = 0,1,2,\ldots,(N-1)$$

$$e^{iQ} = \cos Q + i\sin Q$$

where k represents the subsequent frequency element, N the number of samples, i the square root of the aforementioned equation, Q the sampled signal data, and n the index of the subsequent sample to be processed.

6.6.2 Feature Extraction with MFCC

Mel Frequency Cepstrum Coefficients (MFCC) represent coefficients of a short-time windowed signal, derived through FFT. These coefficients offer improved results compared to time domain operations. MFCC leverages the Mel scale, designed based on human ear sensitivity, making it a popular choice for frequency domain feature extraction in various sound-based applications. The Mel scale aligns with the human ear's sensitivity to sound frequencies up to 1kHz. Mel spectrum involves the application of triangular filters with bandwidth variations corresponding to the Mel scale. A normal frequency E is converted to Mel frequency F as

$$F = 2595\log_{10}\left(\frac{E}{100}+1\right).$$

Moreover, DFT coefficients are examined based on the amplitude frequency response of the Mel filter bank. The amplitude spectrum of the signal is distributed along the Mel scale with equal intervals, each multiplied by the triangular filter. Subsequently, the logarithm of the remaining energy is computed. Since the logarithm of the Mel spectrum coefficients results in real numbers, the discrete cosine transform can be employed to revert to time domain values. These coefficients acquired through this procedure are termed MFCC and can be expressed as

$$M_n = \sum_{k=1}^{L}\left(\log S_k\right)\cos\left[n\left(k-\frac{1}{2}\right)\frac{\pi}{L}\right]$$

where S_k represents the Mel spectrum coefficients. Figure 6.22 shows some MFCC for a sample audio speech from the audio speech clip shown in Figure 6.21.

6.6.3 Emotion Modelling

Neural Structured Learning (NSL) is a deep learning approach that concentrates on training neural networks by incorporating structured signals alongside input features. As introduced in [80], these structured signals are employed to regularize neural network training, encouraging accurate predictions by minimizing supervised loss. Simultaneously, it strives to maintain input structural similarity by minimizing neighbor loss. This approach is versatile and applicable to various neural architectures like standard Feed-forward neural networks, CNN, and RNN. In NSL, training samples are augmented to include structured signals, and, if not explicitly provided, these signals are either constructed or induced through adversarial learning. Subsequently, the augmented training samples, comprising both original and neighboring samples, are input into the neural network to compute their embeddings. The distance between the embedding of a sample and its neighbor is determined and utilized as the neighbor loss, treated as a regularization term and later added to

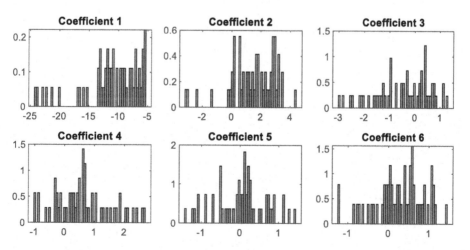

FIGURE 6.22   MFCC coefficients of a sample audio speech.

the final loss. It's noteworthy that, during explicit neighbor-based regularization, any layer of the neural network may be employed to compute the neighbor loss.

6.6.4 Experiments and Results

An audio speech database was compiled for this study, encompassing four expressions, neutral, anger, happy, and sad, totalling 339 audio clips, each lasting around 2 seconds. Employing five-fold cross-validation for experiments, the results are summarized in Table 6.4. Figure 6.23 illustrates the characteristics of the CNN model based on epochs. Additionally, LSTM-based experiments were conducted, achieving a mean recognition rate of 0.88, demonstrating superior performance compared to CNN. The mean recognition rates for all folds corresponding to emotions are 0.94, 0.90, 0.71, and 0.94, respectively. Figure 6.24 showcases the characteristics of the LSTM-based RNN model based on epochs.

TABLE 6.4   The Mean Recall Rates of the Emotions for All the Folds Using Different Approaches

Emotion/Model	CNN	LSTM	NSL
Neutral	0.93	0.88	0.92
Angry	0.91	0.93	0.95
Happy	0.71	0.84	0.86
Sad	0.94	0.8	0.96
Mean	**0.87**	**0.88**	**0.93**

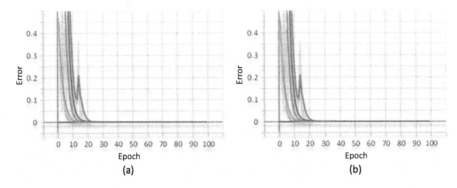

FIGURE 6.23   (a) Loss and (b) accuracy of the CNN model for 100 epochs.

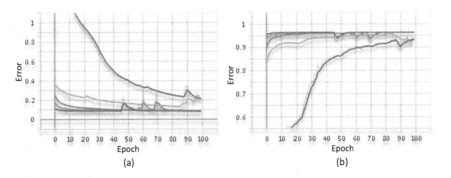

FIGURE 6.24   (a) Loss and (b) accuracy of the LSTM model for 100 epochs.

Finally, NSL-based experiments were executed, yielding a mean recognition rate of 0.93, the highest among all approaches. The mean recognition rates for all folds corresponding to emotions are 0.92, 0.95, 0.85, and 0.97, respectively. Figure 6.25 illustrates the characteristics of the NSL model based on epochs. Figures 6.26–6.28 depict confusion matrices for CNN, LSTM, and NSL, respectively.

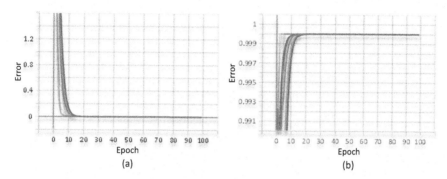

FIGURE 6.25   (a) Loss and (b) accuracy of the NSL model for 100 epochs.

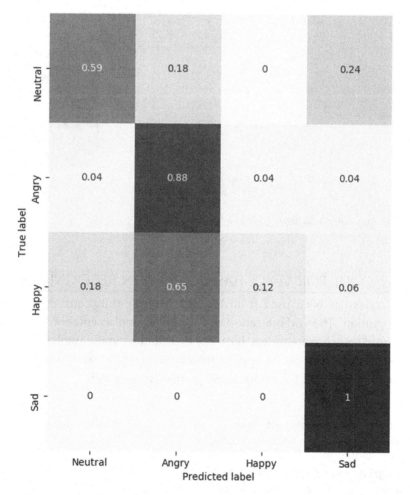

FIGURE 6.26   Confusion matrix using CNN on the dataset.

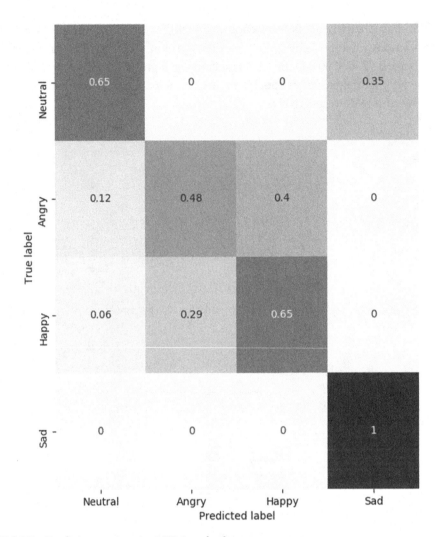

FIGURE 6.27 Confusion matrix using LSTM on the dataset.

6.7 SAMPLE CODE FOR VOICE-BASED EMOTION RECOGNITION

Most of the codes has been used from the link https://github.com/hkveeranki/speech-emotion-recognition. The GitHub repository has basic implementation CNN and LSTM for MFCC-based speech recognition. It can be extended for more implementation such as NSL, CNN+LSTM, etc and can be applied with tensorboard to show different things. The following code is using NSL for emotion recognition from speech.

```
"""
This example demonstrates how to use `LSTM` model from
`speechemotionrecognition` package
"""
import matplotlib.pyplot as plt
from common import extract_data
```

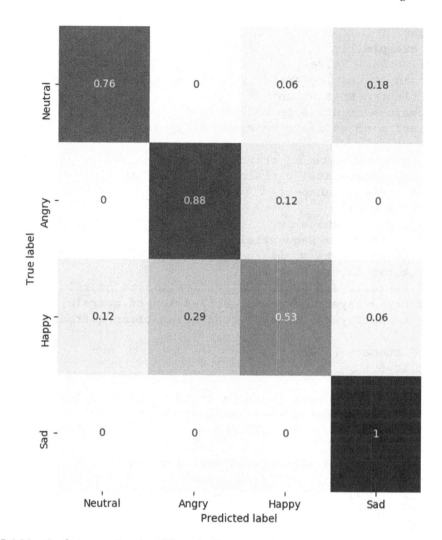

FIGURE 6.28   Confusion matrix using NSL on the dataset.

```
#from speechemotionrecognition.dnn import LSTM
from speechemotionrecognition.utilities import
get_feature_vector_from_mfcc
from datetime import datetime
from packaging import version
import keras
import neural_structured_learning as nsl
import tensorflow as tf
import numpy as np
import pandas as pd
from sklearn.model_selection import KFold
from sklearn.metrics import classification_report,
confusion_matrix
import seaborn as sns
import io
```

```python
import csv
def nsl_example():
    to_flatten = False
    x_train, x_test, y_train, y_test, num_labels = extract_data(
        flatten=to_flatten)
    #y_train = np_utils.to_categorical(y_train)
    #y_test = np_utils.to_categorical(y_test)

    X = np.concatenate([x _ train, x _ test], axis=0)
    Y = np.concatenate([y_train, y_test],    axis=0)
  print(X.shape, Y.shape)
    # create model
    h,w,l=x_train.shape
    model = tf.keras.Sequential([
      tf.keras.Input((w, 1), name='feature'),
      tf.keras.layers.Flatten(),
      tf.keras.layers.Dense(128, activation=tf.nn.relu),
      tf.keras.layers.Dense(64, activation=tf.nn.relu),
      tf.keras.layers.Dense(4, activation=tf.nn.softmax)
        ])
    model.summary()
    n_split=5
    cvscores = []
    for train_index,test_index in KFold(n_split).split(X):
        x_train,x_test=X[train_index],X[test_index]
        y_train,y_test=Y[train_index],Y[test_index]
        scores= []
        adv_config = nsl.configs.make_adv_reg_
config(multiplier=0.1, adv_step_size=0.1)
        adv_model = nsl.keras.AdversarialRegularization(model,
adv_config=adv_config)
    # Compile, train, and evaluate.
        adv_model.compile(optimizer='adam',loss='sparse_
categorical_crossentropy', metrics=['accuracy'])
        logdir=".\\nsllogs4\\fit\\"   +
datetime.now().strftime("%Y%m%d-%H%M%S")
        file_writer = tf.summary.create_file_writer(".\\nsllogs4\\
cm\\"   + datetime.now().strftime("%Y%m%d-%H%M%S"))

        def log _ confusion _ matrix(epoch, logs):
        # Use the model to predict the values from the validation
dataset.
            y_pred=model.predict_classes(x_test)
            con_mat = tf.math.confusion_matrix(labels=y_test,
predictions=y_pred).numpy()
            con_mat_norm = np.around(con_mat.astype('float') /
con_mat.sum(axis=1)[:, np.newaxis], decimals=2)
            classes = ['Neutral', 'Angry', 'Happy', 'Sad']
            con_mat_df = pd.DataFrame(con_mat_norm,index =
classes,columns = classes)
```

```
        figure = plt.figure(figsize=(8, 8))
        sns.heatmap(con_mat_df, annot=True,cmap=plt.cm.Blues)

        #plt.tight _ layout()
        plt.ylabel('True label')
        plt.xlabel('Predicted label')
        buf = io.BytesIO()
        plt.savefig(buf, format='png')
        plt.close(figure)
        buf.seek(0)
        image = tf.image.decode_png(buf.getvalue(),
channels=4)

        image = tf.expand_dims(image, 0)
        # Log the confusion matrix as an image summary.
        with file_writer.as_default():
            tf.summary.image("Confusion Matrix", image,
step=epoch)

        row = ['Info of new split']
        with open(".\\nsllogs4\\nsl.csv", 'a') as csvFile:
            writer = csv.writer(csvFile,  delimiter=",")
            writer.writerows(row)
            writer.writerows(con_mat)
            writer.writerows(con_mat_norm)


    model.summary()

    tensorboard_callback = tf.keras.callbacks.
TensorBoard(log_dir=logdir)
    #cm_callback = keras.callbacks.LambdaCallback(on_epoch_
begin=None, on_epoch_end=log_confusion_matrix,on_batch_begin=None,
on_batch_end=None, on_train_begin=None, on_train_end=None,
**kwargs)
    cm_callback = tf.keras.callbacks.LambdaCallback
(on_epoch_end=log_confusion_matrix)
    adv_model.fit({'feature': x_train, 'label': y_train},
batch_size=20, epochs=100, verbose=0,callbacks=[tensorboard_
callback, cm_callback])

    scores = adv _ model.evaluate({'feature': x _ test, 'label':
y _ test}, verbose=0)
    print("%.2f%%" % scores[2])
    cvscores.append(scores[2] * 100)
    target_names = ['Neutral', 'Angry', 'Happy', 'Sad']
    y_pred=model.predict_classes(x_test)

    print(classification_report(y_test,y_pred,
target_names=target_names))
```

```
    print("%.2f%% (+/- %.2f%%)" % (np.mean(cvscores),
np.std(cvscores)))


#finish Evaluation
if __name__ == '__main__':
    nsl_example()
```

We can change the model part in the above code and apply other models such as CNN+LSTM as bellow:

```
model = Sequential()
    model.add(Conv1D(filters,
                kernel_size,
                padding='valid',
                activation='relu',
                strides=1, input_shape=x_train[0].shape))
    model.add(MaxPooling1D(pool_size=pool_size))
    model.add(LSTM(25, input_shape=x_train[0].shape))
    model.add(Dense(4))
    model.add(Activation('softmax'))
    model.compile(loss='categorical_crossentropy',
            optimizer='adam',
            metrics=['accuracy'])
```

6.8 CONCLUSION

This chapter gave a thorough exploration of image- and audio-based machine learning for emotion recognition. Initially, RGB and depth image-based features have been focused with various machine learning algorithms. A cutting-edge method, LDSP, was employed for real-time emotion recognition through feature extraction. Demonstrations using Python codes showcased different machine learning approaches on a public dataset. Additionally, a sample code illustrated real-time emotion recognition using images from typical RGB color cameras and pre-trained machine learning weights. Brief insights into explainable artificial intelligence results were also provided. Shifting focus to another modality, audio-based emotion recognition was explored. Mel-Frequency Cepstral Coefficients (MFCC) features were tested with diverse machine learning methods, including Recurrent Neural Networks (RNNs), Long Short-Term Memory networks (LSTMs), and Neural Structured Learning (NSL). A Python code example demonstrated the application of MFCC features and various machine learning methods for audio-based emotion recognition.

REFERENCES

[1] A. Shrivastava, D. Dubey, M. Verma, and H. Verma, "Facial Emotion Recognition using Video and Audio," *International Journal of Research Publication and Reviews*, vol. 5, no. 1, pp. 2517–2527, 2024, doi: 10.55248/gengpi.5.0124.0261

[2] M. Z. Uddin, "A depth video-based facial expression recognition system utilizing generalized local directional deviation-based binary pattern feature discriminant analysis," *Multimedia Tools and Applications*, 2015, doi: 10.1007/s11042-015-2614-5

[3] M. H. Prasad and P. Swarnalatha, "Human Emotion Recognition in Video Data Using Deep Learning Frameworks," *Research Square*, vol. 1, pp. 1–10, Jun. 2022, doi: 10.21203/rs.3.rs-1729939/v1

[4] N. Hajarolasvadi, E. Bashirov, and H. Demirel, "Video-based person-dependent and person-independent facial emotion recognition," *Signal, Image and Video Processing*, vol. 15, no. 5, pp. 1049–1056, 2021, doi: 10.1007/s11760-020-01830-0

[5] G. Donato, M. S. Bartlett, J. C. Hagar, P. Ekman, T. J. Sejnowski, "Classifying Facial Actions", *IEEE Transaction on Pattern Analysis and Machine Intelligence*, vol. 21, no. 10, pp. 974–989, 1999.

[6] B. Fasel and J. Luettin, "Recognition of Asymmetric Facial Action Unit Activities and Intensities," in: *Proceedings of the 15th International Conference on Pattern Recognition*, vol. 1, pp. 1100–1103, 2000.

[7] M. Meulders, P. D. Boeck, I. V. Mechelen, and A. Gelman, "Probabilistic Feature Analysis of Facial Perception of Emotions," *Applied Statistics*, vol. 54, no. 4, pp. 781–793, 2005.

[8] A. J. Calder, A. M. Burton, P. Miller, A. W. Young, S. Akamatsu, "A Principal Component Analysis of Facial Expressions," *Vision Research*, vol. 41, pp. 1179–1208, 2001.

[9] S. Dubuisson, F. Davoine, and M. Masson, "A Solution for Facial Expression Representation and Recognition," *Signal Processing: Image Communication*, vol. 17, pp. 657–673, 2002.

[10] I. Buciu, C. Kotropoulos, and I. Pitas, "ICA and Gabor Representation for Facial Expression Recognition", in: *Proceedings of the Conference on Image Processing*, pp. 855–858, 2003.

[11] F. Chen and K. Kotani, "Facial Expression Recognition by Supervised Independent Component Analysis Using MAP Estimation," *IEICE Transactions on Information and Systems*, vol. E91-D, no. 2, pp. 341–350, 2008.

[12] K. Keun-Chang and W. Pedrycz, "Face Recognition Using an Enhanced Independent Component Analysis Approach," *IEEE Transactions on Neural Networks*, vol. 18, no. 2, pp. 530–541, 2007.

[13] Y. Karklin and M. S. Lewicki, "Learning Higher-Order Structures in Natural Images," *Network: Computation in Neural Systems*, vol. 14, pp. 483–499, 2003.

[14] S. -R. Zhou and X. -M. Liang, "Facial Expression Recognition Algorithm Fused ICA and Support Vector Clustering," *Journal of Computer Applications*, vol. 31, no. 6, pp. 1605–1608, 2012.

[15] C. Chao-Fa and F. Y. Shin, "Recognizing Facial Action Units Using Independent Component Analysis and Support Vector Machine," *Pattern Recognition*, vol. 39, pp. 1795–1798, 2006.

[16] X. Wang, X. Huang, and X. Wang, "Face Recognition Using FastICA Algorithm," in: *Proceedings of the International Conference on Control, Automation and Systems Engineering (CASE)*, 2011, pp. 1–4.

[17] X. H. Zhang, Z. F. Liu, Y. J. Guo, and L. Q. Zhao, "Selective Facial Expression Recognition Using fastICA," *Advanced Materials Research*, vol. 433–440, pp. 2755–2761, 2012.

[18] M. S. Bartlett, J. R. Movellan, T. J. Sejnowski, "Face Recognition by Independent Component Analysis," *IEEE Transaction on Neural Networks*, vol. 13, no. 6, pp.1450–1464, 2002.

[19] C. Liu, "Enhanced Independent Component Analysis and Its Application to Content Based Face Image Retrieval," *IEEE Transactions on Systems, Man, and Cybernetics-Part B: Cybernetics*, vol. 34, no. 2, pp. 1117–1127, 2004.

[20] Z. Qiang, C. Chen, Z. Changjun, and W. Xiaopeng, "Independent Component Analysis of Gabor Features for Facial Expression Recognition," in: *Proceedings of the International Symposium on Information Science and Engineering*, 2008, pp. 291–299.

[21] Md. Z. Uddin, W. Khaksar, and J. Torresen, "Facial Expression Recognition Using Salient Features and Convolutional Neural Network," *IEEE Access*, vol. 5, pp. 26146–26161, 2017, doi: 10.1109/access.2017.2777003

[22] T. Ojala, M. Pietikäinen, and T. Mäenpää, "Multiresolution Gray Scale and Rotation Invariant Texture Analysis with Local Binary Patterns," *IEEE Transactions on Pattern Analysis and Machine Intelligence*, vol. 24, pp. 971–987, 2002.

[23] C. Shan, S. Gong, and P. McOwan, "Robust Facial Expression Recognition Using Local Binary Patterns," in: *Proceedings of the IEEE International Conference on Image Processing*, pp. 370–373, 2005.

[24] C. Shan, S. Gong, and P. McOwan, "Facial Expression Recognition Based on Local Binary Patterns: A Comprehensive Study," *Image and Vision Computing*, vol. 27, pp. 803–816, 2009.

[25] T. Jabid, M. H. Kabir, and O. Chae, "Local Directional Pattern (LDP): A Robust Image Descriptor for Object Recognition," in: *Proceedings of the IEEE International Conference on Advanced Video and Signal Based Surveillance*, 2010, pp. 482–487.

[26] M. Z. Uddin, M. M. Hassan, A. Almogren, A. Alamri, M. Alrubaian, and G. Fortino, "Facial Expression Recognition Utilizing Local Direction-Based Robust Features and Deep Belief Network," *IEEE Access*, vol 5, pp. 4525–4536, 2017.

[27] H. M. Ebied, "Feature Extraction Using PCA and Kernel-PCA for Face Recognition," in: *Proceedings of the 8th International Conference on Informatics and Systems (INFOS)*, 2017, pp. 72–77.

[28] F. Yaghouby, A. Ayatollahi, and R. Soleimani, "Classification of Cardiac Abnormalities Using Reduced Features of Heart Rate Variability Signal," *World Applied Sciences Journal*, vol. 6, no. 11, pp. 1547–1554, 2009.

[29] I. Cohen, N. Sebe, A. Garg, L. S. Chen, and T. S. Huang, "Facial Expression Recognition from Video Sequences: Temporal and Static Modeling," *Computer Vision and Image Understanding*, vol. 91, pp. 160–187, 2003.

[30] S. Kiranyaz, T. Ince, and M. Gabbouj, "Real-Time Patient-Specific ECG Classification by 1-D Convolutional Neural Networks," *IEEE Transactions on Biomedical Engineering*, vol. 63, no. 3, pp. 664–675, 2016.

[31] G. E. Hinton, S. Osindero, Y. -W. Teh, "A Fast Learning Algorithm for Deep Belief Nets," *Neural Computation*, vol. 18, no. 7, pp. 1527–1554, 2006.

[32] F. Deboeverie, S. Roegiers, G. Allebosch, P. Veelaert, and W. Philips, "Human gesture classification by brute-force machine learning for exergaming in physiotherapy," in: *Proceedings of IEEE Conference on Computational Intelligence and Games (CIG)*, Santorini, 2016, pp. 1–7.

[33] A. Mollahosseini, D. Chan, and M. H. Mahoor, "Going deeper in facial expression recognition using deep neural networks," in: *Proceedings of the IEEE Winter Conference on Applications of Computer Vision (WACV)*, 2016, pp. 1–10.

[34] M. Liu, S. Li, S. Shan, and X. Chen, "AU-Aware Deep Networks for Facial Expression Recognition," in: *Proceedings of the 10th IEEE International Conference and Workshops on Automatic Face and Gesture Recognition (FG)*, 2013, pp. 1–6.

[35] Z. Yu and C. Zhang, "Image Based Static Facial Expression Recognition with Multiple Deep Network Learning," in: *Proceedings of the ACM on International Conference on Multimodal Interaction*, 2015, pp. 435–442.

[36] P. Liu, S. Han, Z. Meng, and Y. Tong, "Facial Expression Recognition via a Boosted Deep Belief Network," in: *Proceedings of the IEEE Conference on Computer Vision and Pattern Recognition*, 2014, pp.1805–1812.

[37] O. Oreifej and Z. Liu, "Hon4d: Histogram of Oriented 4d Normals for Activity Recognition from Depth Sequences," in: *Proceedings of the IEEE Conference on Computer Vision and Pattern Recognition*, 2013, pp. 716–723.

[38] A. Vieira, E. Nascimento, G. Oliveira, Z. Liu, and M. Campos, "Stop: Space-Time Occupancy Patterns for 3d Action Recognition from Depth Map Sequences," in: *Proceedings of the Progress in Pattern Recognition, Image Analysis, Computer Vision, and Applications*, 2012, pp. 252–259.

[39] J. Sung, C. Ponce, B. Selman, and A. Saxena, "Unstructured Human Activity Detection from RGBD Images," in: *Proceedings of the IEEE International Conference on Robotics and Automation*, 2012, pp. 842–849.

[40] Y. Tian, T. Kanade, and J. Cohn, "Evaluation of Gabor Wavelet Based Facial Action Unit Recognition in Image Sequences of Increasing Complexity," in: *Proceedings of the Fifth IEEE International Conference on Automatic Face and Gesture Recognition*, 2002, pp. 229–234.

[41] N. A. Savran, H. Dibeklioğlu, O. Çeliktutan, B. Gökberk, B. Sankur, and L. Akarun, "Bosphorus Database for 3D Face Analysis," in: *Proceedings of the First COST 2101 Workshop on Biometrics and Identity Management (BIOID 2008)*, Roskilde University, Denmark, 7–9 May.

[42] B. S. Savran and M. T. Bilge, "Comparative Evaluation of 3D versus 2D Modality for Automatic Detection of Facial Action Units," *Pattern Recognition*, vol. 45, no. 2, pp. 767–782, 2012.

[43] B. S. Savran and M. T. Bilge, "Regression-Based Intensity Estimation of Facial Action Units," *Image and Vision Computing*, vol. 30, no. 10, pp. 774–784, 2012.

[44] P. Baxter and J. G. Trafton, "Cognitive Architectures for Human-Robot Interaction," in: *Proceedings of the 2014 ACM/IEEE International Conference on Human–Robot Interaction – HRI '14*, Bielefeld, Germany: ACM Press, 2014, pp. 504–505.

[45] S. Tadeusz, "Application of Vision Information to Planning Trajectories of Adept Six-300 Robot," in: *Proceedings of 21st International Conference on Methods and Models in Automation and Robotics (MMAR)*, Miedzyzdroje, Poland, 2016, pp. 1069–1075.

[46] Y. U. Sonmez and A. Varol, "New Trends in Speech Emotion Recognition," in: *2019 7th International Symposium on Digital Forensics and Security (ISDFS)*, Jun. 2019.

[47] T. Ozseven, "Investigation of the Effect of Spectrogram Images and Different Texture Analysis Methods on Speech Emotion Recognition," *Applied Acoustics*, vol. 142, pp. 70–77, 2018.

[48] H. O. Nasereddin and A. R. Omari, "Classification Techniques for Automatic Speech Recognition (ASR) Algorithms used with Real Time Speech Translation," in: *Computing Conference*, 2017, pp. 200–207.

[49] K. Tarunika, R. B. Pradeeba, and P. Aruna, "Applying Machine Learning Techniques for Speech Emotion Recognition," in: *9th International Conference On Computing Communication and Networking Technologies (ICCCNT)*, 10–12 July. 2018.

[50] S. Prasomphan, "Improvement Of Speech Emotion Recognition with Neural Network Classifier by Using Speech Spectrogram," in: *2015 International Conference on Systems Signals and Image Processing (IWSSIP)*, 10–12 September, 2015, pp. 72–76.

[51] H. Zhao, N. Ye, and R. Wang, "A Survey on Automatic Emotion Recognition Using Audio Big Data and Deep Learning Architectures," in: *2018 IEEE 4th International Conference on Big Data Security on Cloud (BigDataSecurity), IEEE International Conference on High Performance and Smart Computing, (HPSC) and IEEE International Conference on Intelligent Data and Security (IDS)*, May 2018.

[52] G. Trigeorgis, F. Ringeval, R. Brueckner, E. Marchi, M. A. Nicolaou, B. Schuller, and S. Zafeiriou, "Adieu Features? End-to-End Speech Emotion Recognition Using a Deep Convolutional Recurrent Network," in: *IEEE International Conference on Acoustics, Speech and Signal Processing*, 2016.

[53] D. Tang, P. Kuppens, L. Geurts, and T. van Waterschoot, "End-to-end speech emotion recognition using a novel context-stacking dilated convolution neural network," *EURASIP Journal on Audio, Speech, and Music Processing*, vol. 2021, no. 1, May 2021, doi: 10.1186/s13636-021-00208-5

[54] G. Liu, S. Cai, and C. Wang, "Speech Emotion Recognition Based on Emotion Perception," *EURASIP Journal on Audio, Speech, and Music Processing*, vol. 2023, no. 1, May 2023, doi: 10.1186/s13636-023-00289-4

[55] M. Fujimoto, "Factored Deep Convolutional Neural Networks for Noise Robust Speech Recognition," in: *Proceedings of Interspeech*, Aug. 2017, pp. 3837–3841.

[56] T. Sivanagaraja, M. K. Ho, A. W. H. Khong, and Y. Wang, "End-to-End Speech Emotion Recognition Using Multi-Scale Convolution Networks," *2017 Asia-Pacific Signal and Information Processing Association Annual Summit and Conference (APSIPA ASC)*, Dec. 2017.

[57] D. Le and E. M. Provost, "Emotion Recognition from Spontaneous Speech Using Hidden Markov Models with Deep Belief Networks," in: *2013 IEEE Workshop on Automatic Speech Recognition and Understanding*, Dec. 2013.

[58] G. E. Hinton, S. Osindero, and Y. The, "A Fast Learning Algorithm for Deep Belief Nets," *Neural Computation*, vol. 18, no. 7, pp. 1527–1554, 2006.

[59] A. Fischer and C. Igel "Training Restricted Boltzmann Machines: An Introduction," *Pattern Recognition*, vol. 47, no. 1, pp. 25–39, 2014.

[60] B.M. Asl, S.K. Setarehdan, and M. Mohebbi, "Support Vector Machine-Based Arrhythmia Classification Using Reduced Features of Heart Rate Variability Signal," *Artificial Intelligence in Medicine*, vol. 44, pp. 51–64, 2008.

[61] M. Z. Uddin, "A Depth Video-Based Facial Expression Recognition System Utilizing Generalized Local Directional Deviation-Based Binary Pattern Feature Discriminant Analysis," *Multimedia Tools and Applications*, vol. 75, no. 12, pp. 6871–6886, 2016.

[62] M. Z. Uddin, W. Khaksar, and J. Torresen, "Facial Expression Recognition Using Salient Features and Convolutional Neural Network," *IEEE Access*, vol. 5, pp. 26146–26161, 2017.

[63] W Li., Z. Zhang, and Z. Liu, "Expandable Data-Driven Graphical Modeling of Human Actions Based on Salient Postures," *IEEE Transactions on Circuits and Systems for Video Technology*, vol. 18, no. 11, pp. 1499–1510, 2008.

[64] J. Wang, Z. Liu, J. Chorowski, Z. Chen, and Y. Wu, " Robust 3d Action Recognition with Random Occupancy Patterns," in: *European Conference on Computer Vision*, 2012, pp. 872–885.

[65] X. Yang, C. Zhang, and Y Tian, "Recognizing Actions Using Depth Motion Maps-based Histograms of Oriented Gradients," in: *ACM International Conference on Multimedia*, 2012, pp. 1057–1060.

[66] M. Z. Uddin, M. M. Hassan, A. Alsanad, and C. Savaglio, "A Body Sensor Data Fusion and Deep Recurrent Neural Network-Based Behavior Recognition Approach for Robust Healthcare," *Information Fusion*, vol. 55, pp. 105–115, 2020.

[67] "Neural Structured Learning: Training with Structured Signals," Tensorflow. Available: https://www.tensorflow.org/neural_structured_learning/. [Accessed: 06-Jan-2020].

[68] T. D. Bui, S. Ravi, and V. Ramavajjala, "Neural Graph Learning," in: *Proceedings of the Eleventh ACM International Conference on Web Search and Data Mining – WSDM '18*, 2018.

[69] H. H. Aghdam, E. J. Heravi, and D. Puig, "Explaining Adversarial Examples by Local Properties of Convolutional Neural Networks," in: *Proceedings of the 12th International Joint Conference on Computer Vision, Imaging and Computer Graphics Theory and Applications*, 2017.

[70] M. Uddin, W. Khaksar, and J. Torresen, "Ambient Sensors for Elderly Care and Independent Living: A Survey," *Sensors*, vol. 18, no. 7, p. 2027, 2018.

[71] A. Fleury, N. Noury, M. Vacher, H. Glasson, and J. -F. Seri, "Sound and speech detection and classification in a Health Smart Home," in: *2008 30th Annual International Conference of the IEEE Engineering in Medicine and Biology Society*, Aug. 2008, pp. 4644–4647.

[72] Y. Li, Z. Zeng, M. Popescu, and K. C. Ho, "Acoustic Fall Detection Using a Circular Microphone Array," in: *2010 Annual International Conference of the IEEE Engineering in Medicine and Biology*, Aug. 2010, pp. 2242–2245.

[73] Yun Li, M. Popescu, K. C. Ho, and D. P. Nabelek, "Improving Acoustic Fall Recognition by Adaptive Signal Windowing," in: *2011 Annual International Conference of the IEEE Engineering in Medicine and Biology Society*, Aug. 2011, pp. 7589–7592.

[74] Y. Li, K. C. Ho, and M. Popescu, "A Microphone Array System for Automatic Fall Detection," *IEEE Transactions on Biomedical Engineering*, vol. 59, no. 5, pp. 1291–1301, 2012.

[75] M. Popescu, Y. Li, M. Skubic, and M. Rantz, "An Acoustic Fall Detector System that Uses Sound Height Information to Reduce the False Alarm Rate," in: *2008 30th Annual International Conference of the IEEE Engineering in Medicine and Biology Society*, Aug. 2008, pp. 4628–4631.

[76] M. Popescu and A. Mahnot, "Acoustic Fall Detection Using One-Class Classifiers," in: *2009 Annual International Conference of the IEEE Engineering in Medicine and Biology Society*, Sep. 2009, pp. 3505–3508.

[77] M. Vacher, D. Istrate, F. Portet, T. Joubert, T. Chevalier, S. Smidtas, B. Meillon, B. Lecouteux, M. Sehili, P. Chahuara, and S. Meniard, "The Sweet-Home Project: Audio Technology in Smart Homes to Improve Well-Being and Reliance," in: *2011 Annual International Conference of the IEEE Engineering in Medicine and Biology Society*, Aug. 2011, pp. 5291–5294.

[78] X. Zhuang, J. Huang, G. Potamianos, and M. Hasegawa-Johnson, "Acoustic Fall Detection Using Gaussian Mixture Models and GMM Supervectors," in: *2009 IEEE International Conference on Acoustics, Speech and Signal Processing*, Apr. 2009, pp. 69–72.

[79] L. Zhang, S. Walter, Xueyao Ma, P. Werner, A. Al-Hamadi, H. C. Traue, and S. Gruss, "'BioVid Emo DB': A Multimodal Database for Emotion Analyses Validated by Subjective Ratings," in: *2016 IEEE Symposium Series on Computational Intelligence (SSCI)*, Dec. 2016.

[80] Md. Z. Uddin and E. G. Nilsson, "Emotion Recognition Using Speech and Neural Structured Learning to Facilitate Edge Intelligence," *Engineering Applications of Artificial Intelligence*, vol. 94, p. 103775, 2020, doi: 10.1016/j.engappai.2020.103775

Index

Pages in *italics* refer to figures and pages in **bold** refer to tables.

Printed in the United States
by Baker & Taylor Publisher Services